RAPID NOVEL

A QUICK GUIDE TO WRITING A 50,000-WORD
NOVEL IN 5 DAYS

JEWEL ALLEN

Rapid Novel
Copyright © 2022 Jewel P. Allen
Cover and interior design: Jewel P. Allen
Stock vector cover photo: Depositphotos
First publication: November 2022

No part of this book may be used, reproduced, or transmitted in any manner without written permission, except in the case of brief quotations for critical articles and reviews. All rights reserved.

∼

Special thanks to my sprinting friends for sticking with me through those all-day sprints. As always, my husband for your love and patience and not taking me too much to task for disappearing into my office while on book deadline. Last but not the least, my Heavenly Father for giving me the opportunity to create stories.

Join my Rapid Releasers group on Facebook.
Check out my Rapid Release series under Jewel P. Allen and my novels under Jewel Allen.

Get my free, downloadable *50K to 5 Days Novel Planner* at
www.JewelAllen.com/get-a-free-book

CONTENTS

Rapid Novel Summary	1
Introduction	3
1. Why write a novel in 5 days?	5
2. My Journey to 50K	7
3. What is a "quality" draft?	12
4. A little back story	14
5. Getting past the fear	16
6. Choosing your project	18
7. Prepping: If you have one day or more	21
8. Prepping: If you have an hour	25
9. Using an Outline	27
10. Understanding your characters	31
11. 50K in 5 Days Schedule	33
12. When Life Happens	36
13. Writing Characters with Depth	39
14. How to up your word count	41
15. Recording your word count	45
16. Self-Care	46
17. Rest and Recharge	48
18. Start your story	50
19. How to fix a sucky opening (without trashing the whole thing)	52
20. Making your story flow	54
21. Making your words count	57
22. K-Drama your way to a fabulous novel	59
23. How to Fix a Franken-Plot	61
24. Shoring up the Middle Sag	63
25. Stick to It	66
26. Finish strong	68
27. After the 50K	70

28. Parting Thoughts 73
29. Bonus: Word Count Tracker 75

RAPID NOVEL SUMMARY

Perhaps you are writing your first novel. Or want to write a 50,000-word novel in 30 days for National Novel Writing Month (NaNoWriMo)*, or a similar writing challenge. Maybe you are already an experienced novelist wanting to up your speed and efficiency in drafting your novels to meet your deadlines and build your backlist.

In this short, no-fluff, instantly actionable guide, Jewel Allen shares her method for writing a 50,000-word novel in 5 days. Even for pantsers without tons of pre-planning, applying this technique can result in a clean, finished draft that would require minimal revisions, and ultimately, could be self-published within 30 days.

*This book is not affiliated with NaNoWriMo, though I am a huge fan and endorse it highly. I owe NaNoWriMo the kick in the pants I needed to unlock me from paralysis and start my career as a self-published author.

. . .

**Someone asked if the material here is the shortened version of tips I put in my 2019 book *Rapid Release*. Some of the principles will resurface here. *Rapid Novel* includes new, more efficient techniques I've learned and personally tested from subsequent years rapid releasing.

INTRODUCTION

It's 2022 and I had just won NaNoWriMo (National Novel Writing Month) early in the wee hours of Day 5. "Winning" meant I had written 50,000 words, a completed novel that had been on my backburner for the past three years.

On Day 1, I started at 10 p.m. On Day 5, I ended at 1:38 a.m. My author friends asked me for my secrets to writing a book in 5 days. As I shared my advice in batches of posts, it soon became apparent I needed to write a book to add to my Rapid Release series.

There are two ways of writing a novel for a writing challenge like NaNoWriMo.

One is to get words any which way you can, no matter if it's a tangled mess of a book/s afterward. My first NaNoWriMo project, a 50,000-word historical novel, was like this. It took me a few months to revise, but at least I had something to work with. You could also write a series of novellas whose word count add up to 50,000. I've known some writers who count blog posts. Which, I suppose, is fine. 50,000 words is 50,000 words.

The second way, which I will talk about throughout in

this book, is writing 50,000 words towards a novel that is complete or close to complete, will require minimal revisions, and ultimately could be self-published within 30 days. My most recent NaNoWriMo project, *Billionaire Bunker,* falls under this category. So have several of my books where I've procrastinated and I find myself having 3 to 5 days before I have to get the document to my editor.

Rapid Novel will lay out, in detail, the process I've used over the decade or so I have participated in NaNoWriMo, as well as rapid releasing 40+ novels.

This book will show how you, too, can write a 50,000-word novel in 5 days.

1

WHY WRITE A NOVEL IN 5 DAYS?

NaNoWriMo gives a writer 30 days to complete a manuscript, which is perfectly reasonable, because . . . life. So yes, I recognize that this book is NaNo on steroids. It means that at a minimum to get 50K words in 5 days, one must write a daily average of 10K words.

Why 5 days, Jewel, you ask? Well . . . writing fast gets you in the "zone," your story will feel more dynamic, and you will be able to keep the style more consistent. Plus, you'll get to "The End" faster!

So how does one go from writing 1,667 words per day to 17,368? This book will show you how.

Flashback...

For my first NaNoWriMo project in 2008, I divided the word count I needed to get 50,000. I aimed to get 1,667 words a day. I printed out a calendar and stamped each day I reached my word goal with a red Hello Kitty. I also tied rewards for every so many days I gained a stamp. I made adjustments for Thanksgiving, figuring I would not be getting my word counts around that holiday.

Fourteen years later for my NaNoWriMo project,

Billionaire Bunker, I wrote 2,818 words on Day 1; 11,183 on Day 2; 16,067 on Day 3; 17,368 on Day 4; and 2,679 words on Day 5. Technically speaking, I could have completed the book in 4 days.

So . . . is it possible to write a 50,000-word novel in 5 days? The answer is a resounding yes!

A gentle reminder...

If this is your first attempt at a 50K-word novel, don't be too hard on yourself if you are simply trying to get a minimum daily count. Remember that I reached this milestone by practicing for 14 years, some of the last four of which included rapid releasing 50K-word novels every month. Also, some genres like fantasy, paranormal, or mystery, to mention a few, can require massive world-building, which in turn will require more prep work to avoid time-consuming revisions later.

To sum up, it is possible to increase your speed and efficiency writing a novel, no matter your writing experience. Beginner or advanced, set a personal record, and then try to beat it. Keep setting your sights higher and higher until you, too, can be a writing machine. If you're ready to get to the next level in writing a quality 50,000-word novel in 5 days, read on.

2

MY JOURNEY TO 50K

I stink at hiking.

Once, during a dream safari vacation in Africa, my husband and I went on this fun river-running day expedition down the Zambezi River, the spray of the stupendously grand Victoria Falls forming a mist in the background. Getting down to the rafts was easy. But getting out after the rafting adventure was punishing.

Employees of our river guide service carried parts of our boat up this steep mountain like they weighed nothing while I had to stop at every switchback to catch my breath and let the pounding of my heart subside. The employees asked after me solicitously, even offering to carry me up, but my pride prevented me from saying yes. Towards the top, one of them said I was almost there, and I mustered the strength to finish the hike.

∼

A lot of times as I have drafted a 50,000-word novel in 5 days, I've felt that same way, breathless, in pain, and out of shape. Feeling out of my depth. Wanting to give up so badly with only my prideful refusal to quit shoring me up.

Several points while I wrote *Billionaire Bunker* come to mind. After the bombastic opening when I was feeling good, I realized I had no scientific basis for what was going on in the plot. It was laughable, me, an English-major type, writing about scientists when I couldn't even stand the sight of someone drawing blood from my arm. I went ahead and made things up, even though it felt dumb.

Another time during the sagging middle, I was sure this was the most boring book in the world and why did I even think this plot was going to fly? I switched gears, added a plot twist, and was energized by the change.

Sometimes my body ached from being held in the same position most of the day and I had to physically walk away from my desk to scrounge for Cheetos in the pantry. Sour cream and onion potato chips. Brownies. Leftovers. Anything to relieve the pressure of this grueling, seemingly unending task. Towards the end of an eight-hour writing day, my eyes turned blurry and I almost couldn't see what I'm writing.

And still, I kept on because the story, in its speed and raw power, had seized me by the throat and would not let go. For all the difficulties of writing fast, the story developed like a movie and I couldn't wait to see what would happen next.

At the end of each 10K or more day, my hands cramping and my author body showing its age, I closed my laptop with a little tired sigh, collecting all my things and padding out to the darkness of my house, my husband already in bed. The 10K notches were like switchbacks, reminding me that this torturous journey would eventually end.

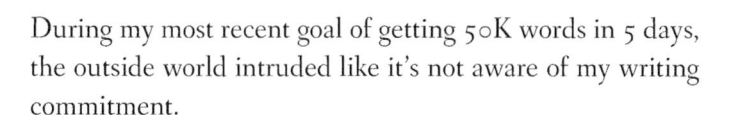

During my most recent goal of getting 50K words in 5 days, the outside world intruded like it's not aware of my writing commitment.

My win with *Billionaire Bunker* came at a particularly busy week. I am a councilwoman for our city. I fielded phone calls from constituents on Day 1. On Day 2, I had a council meeting at 6:30 p.m.. Until the very last, I finally pulled myself away from my story, which had been going well. But I went and as though the gods favored me, the meeting was relatively short. I went back home and started up the typing once again. That was lucky.

Sometimes, however, it's harder to deal with a disruption. November also happens to be the tail end of elections. During my most recent NaNo, someone had included me in a group text which exploded into a major political disagreement. Near tears, I tried to get out of the group, and was able to delete the conversation. But the emotional damage was done. My lower word counts that day reflected my agitated state of mind, and I railed at the world for such toxicity. Luckily, I was able to get through this dark time, pouring my frustration into my plot. I had my main character express all my pent-up emotions as she fought the villain off.

One NaNoWrimo came at the heels of my dad passing away in late October after a ten-year battle with cancer. After his funeral, I wasn't sure if I wanted to, nor should, write a novel. But pushing through only made my victory sweeter, like my dad was watching from heaven above. I imagined that if he could have, he would have bought a dozen copies of my finished book to give away to the nurses who tended to him at his sickbed, like he'd done while still alive.

~

When I cross the 40K threshold, my body leans into the keyboard. I can smell victory, even as I tell myself I shouldn't be so cocky and wait until I have the 50K words in hand. Over the years of my writing novels, it's still the same way each time. I know when I've reached the last stretch. When I know this story might actually be finished and see the light of day.

My word count soars into the 900s consistently and I'm raring to start sprinting again. Sometimes, I even keep writing past the timer. Concluding the story propels me into a frenzied mood, a second wind, if you will, where I draw strength from a reservoir I forget that I have and am capable of, time and time again. This is the power of creating. The allure of that sharp taste of victory as I type The End.

When I did so with *Billionaire Bunker* at 1:38 a.m. and went back to add 5,000 more words to get 50,013 with an official win, I sat at my desk stunned for several minutes. Another story under my belt. Another NaNo win. Another book that I could mold and shape into something better that hopefully others will love as much as I do. And in 5 days no less.

It's that high that draws me to writing a novel again, and again, even if each starting blank page taunts me that I can't do this.

But I can, and I do.

~

After my win with *Billionaire Bunker*, I stepped out of my office, closed the door, and went into our bedroom, where my husband lay, sound asleep. I padded into our bathroom and turned on the light.

I looked at my reflection, noting my haggard face, though it could have been worse. I've finished many a novel when the sun is starting to lighten the horizon. I brushed my teeth and climbed in bed gingerly, trying not to jiggle my sleeping husband, scaring off our jittery cat who doesn't like me, my bones luxuriating in the softness of the mattress.

Unable to resist, I embraced my husband who was faced away from me on his side. I squeezed him close and whispered into the warmth of his back, "I did it! I finished my story."

I've told him this many times in the middle of the night throughout our 30-year marriage, as I have worked as a journalist, and then as an author, and he still sounded like he always does.

In a cheerful, sleepy voice, he held my hand against his chest and said, "Good job."

3

WHAT IS A "QUALITY" DRAFT?

When I aim for a quality, 50,000-word draft in five days, I aim for the following:

- Will not require a lot of rewriting or moving scenes around
- Has beautiful language and description that does not bog down the pacing
- Has fleshed out and believable characters who act consistent to their traits
- Goes deep into themes and reveals my authentic author imprint
- Is not riddled with typos
- Has good pacing, neither too slow nor too fast; just right

Take a minute and answer this question for yourself. What are your quality goals for your novel?

- _____
- _____
- _____
- _____
- _____
- _____

4

A LITTLE BACK STORY

I'D HAD this idea for a billionaire sci-fi series for several years now, since clear back in 2019 when I commissioned 5 series covers. The past NaNoWriMos, however, I chose other projects.

Why?

Because I was scared.

Over the years, I've written novels in different fiction genres: historical and contemporary romance, as well as several tropes: cowboys, billionaire, firefighter, royals. With each pivot, I prepared by reading in the genre and doing my research.

This new series would be post-apocalyptic zombie, leaning sci-fi. My first novel, *Ghost Moon Night*, had zombies, but that is where the similarity ends. Realizing I'd been postponing *Billionaire Bunker* for three years now, I finally girded up my courage and chose to do it. Even though I'd had little time to prepare.

For my 2022 NaNoWriMo project, I went from finishing revisions on a cowboy book to jumping right into *Billionaire Bunker*. I skimmed an outline I'd written years ago but knew I wouldn't stick to it, judging from my eye-rolls. I even ignored some first chapters I'd started here and there, wanting to start afresh. I jotted down series details like character names and physical characteristics. And that was it! Game on.

I joined a writing sprint with other authors, and, despite my shot nerves, started writing.

5

GETTING PAST THE FEAR

When I first immigrated to America from the Philippines some thirty years ago, one of the most interesting experiences for me was going to a water park in Salt Lake City, Utah.

I went on a water slide that seemed pretty high up. I figured it must be fun; the lines were long. My boyfriend-then-husband-now went ahead of me. I sat down on the slide, covered with flowing water. I chuckled because I had to scoot on my swimsuit bottom to get to the edge.

And then boom!

One moment I was on the slide, and the next, I was plunging straight down. The slide was so steep and so tall, I still get clammy hands remembering how I was so shocked I couldn't even scream. I descended for probably what took just seconds but felt like an eternity.

Had I known about the slide's steepness, or seen videos of people going down it, I probably wouldn't have done it. And yet, I was able to do it and survive.

The same goes for writing. Sometimes, we are better off not focusing on what is beyond that blank page, and just plunge right in. It will be the hardest thing, terror will nearly paralyze you, but you will survive.

And when you are looking at the 50K word counter on your document, thinking, *I did that faster than I ever have*, you will feel the greatest rush.

Believe you can do it, and you will.

Writing a novel doesn't even involve death-defying water slides, even if it feels like it. (For the record, I probably would never go down a slide like that again, knowing what I know now.)

Before self-publishing my first novel, I felt sick to my stomach for weeks. It's gotten easier since with each book, but I still stare at a blank page with nausea.

When you've been going along with good daily word counts and then aim higher— 5K, 10K, 17K—fear and doubt will grab you by the throat and scare you back into a corner, thinking, *who am I to try that?*

Ask any writer who produces words at a high daily rate, and they'll say they're no one special. They still procrastinate cleaning the bathroom like everyone else, and their husbands have to tell them to be ready ten minutes earlier than actual departure time because they're always tardy.

But one thing they're real good at is overcoming the fear when it threatens to swallow them, with each goal set higher, and higher, and higher.

Your story won't be perfect? Write anyway.

You might get bad reviews? Write anyway.

You don't have a detailed plan for this novel? Write anyway.

You want this story out fast, don't you? Let that desire and determination carry you through all the negative emotions you might associate with drafting novels. What was past was past. Look to the future.

6

CHOOSING YOUR PROJECT

IT WAS fall of 2021 and the story on National Public Radio transfixed me. I was driving to my daughter's a couple of hours away and I hung on to every word. I even stayed sitting in the parking lot several minutes to make sure I caught it to the end. It was an interview of Paul McCartney by Terry Gross, on All Things Considered.

Paul was on the show to talk about his two-volume collector's item called "The Lyrics: 1956 to the Present" which he launched on November 2. In it, he shares the lyrics he composed while performing with the Beatles, and the inspiration behind them.

For example, he dreamed the melody to "Yesterday." Woke up one morning and ran it past John Lennon to make sure he hadn't just heard it somewhere else. How amazing would that be to dream up a whole melody? And then he wrote the lyrics to fit it.

Which brings me to inspiration for your story. I don't know about you, but I find it hard to choose what story to write for a writing challenge. There are always so many competing ideas in my head, coming at me from everywhere.

If you're still trying to choose what story to write, here are some ideas:

1. If you have a dream, write it down.
2. Read newspaper articles and jot down headlines that catch your attention.
3. Write in a genre you've never written in before.
4. Write a fictional journal entry every day during the month from a character you inherently wouldn't get along with.
5. Pick a setting where you've traveled to or want to travel to.
6. Make up a character who's exactly the opposite of you and have them "tell" you their story in a few paragraphs.
7. Write down your story ideas in a notebook.

One of my NaNo projects was inspired by a ranch cattle branding day I was able to go on late summer this year. And it is a spin-off from side characters in my current cowboy romance series.

I am a firm believer that your novel chooses you. With your unique imprint, you can bring this book out into the world, as only you can. The time and place is now. The stars are aligning. With this in mind, keep yourself open to inspiration.

There are several, equally legitimate, reasons to choose a certain novel as your project. They could be:

1. You love reading in this genre.

2. This is a book you've been scared of writing and it's about time you did.
3. You want to write fast to take advantage of the popularity of a genre.
4. There are no books like this out there and you want to be first.

I've used each of the reasons above in past NaNoWriMo challenges. Whatever the reason, pick your project and lean in.

Challenge: Brainstorm potential stories and pick the one that feels right!

- _____
- _____
- _____
- _____
- _____
- _____

7

PREPPING: IF YOU HAVE ONE DAY OR MORE

NOTE: If you are pressed for time, as in, you needed to start your project last week, or you are literally trying to write your NaNoWriMo project, skim through this or skip to the next chapter. You have my permission. Sometime, when things have settled, go back to this chapter.

∼

A. Prepare for a series

Perhaps you only want to write a standalone. That's fine. Standalones have made bestseller lists since time immemorial. You don't have to write series, if you absolutely don't want to. Just make sure, when you change your mind, you can do so.

Here's food for thought. Have you noticed that bestsellers that seemed to start as standalones often have sequel books or movies soon after? It's a no-brainer. Hook a reader on a book and they will devour the rest of a series so long as you make the series compelling enough. What if your book does well? Do you have a plan to continue it into a series?

Advice on planning a series can take up a whole separate book, but the following section spells out how, in a nutshell. You can either write your series notes in a document or spreadsheet, or, if you are like me, use one of my Series Planners (which I created because I could never keep track of those loose papers and digital documents).

1. Think of your main characters as cogs in a bigger machine. In a romance, that would be the hero and his love interest. What kind of family and upbringing do they have? How did it affect the kind of person they are now? Where do their family members live? Do they have close relationships? There's nothing weirder than a character in a story set around Christmas, for example, and they're not planning on going home or staying away, for instance. Note: A "family" can also be traded for a substitute with common connections, such as work colleagues or friends.
2. World-building is crucial for genres such as fantasy and sci-fi, but it's important for other genres, too. Make a short list of important settings and brainstorm your magic systems. But don't over-plan to the point you're procrastinating on the book.
3. Research your time period, setting or subject. This will lend your writing the authenticity it needs and give you confidence as a writer. As you write, there will be gaps in what you know, and that is okay. I put ## where I encounter a

need for the right word or more research. Someone suggested [} to me because there is no need to press the shift button, because little things like that count in writing fast.
4. Identify your side characters. If they will be leads in future series, give them distinct personality and physical traits. You don't want all of your heroes to be blond and blue-eyed, unless you differentiate them with other characteristics.
5. Choose different tropes for each series book to avoid writing novels too similar to each other. For example, in my Riverdale Ranch Romance cowboy series, I used older brother of best friend, enemies to lovers, secret love, city girl / cowboy, secret identity, grumpy / sunshine and amnesia.

B. Prepare for your book

1. Write a short sentence for each book in the series which identifies its story arc. For example, my blurb for *Billionaire Bunker* reads, a billionaire and his scientist ex race to find a cure for a zombie virus before his billionaire bunker falls in the wrong hands.
2. Read books and watch movies that could inspire your new project. When I was getting ready to write the next installment in my firefighter romance, I watched a couple of firefighter

movies. I love self-help books, but I had to stop listening to an audio book with a heavier theme because the vibe for my project wasn't right.

C. Prepare a loose outline (see Chapter 7, "Using an Outline")

8

PREPPING: IF YOU HAVE AN HOUR

THIS WAS SERIOUSLY ME, this past NaNoWriMo (and, let's face it, with most of my novels).

On Day 1, I had a cowboy romance due to my beta reader and revised it until dinner. After dinner, at around 10 p.m., I was getting my words down for *Billionaire Bunker*.

This is what I did.

1. Don't panic. What good is it to panic anyway? It won't get your novel written.
2. Blurb your story. What is your story about? Identify the main characters, their goals and the obstacles to their goals. Use this like your north star. If you need to change it as you go along, change it. For example, my blurb for *Billionaire Bunker* reads, a billionaire and his scientist ex race to find a cure for a zombie virus before his billionaire bunker falls in the wrong hands.

3. Scribble down the main and side characters' first and last names, picking ones that do not start with the same letter, to avoid confusion.
4. Note these basic but important info somewhere for each main and side character. Trust me, it will save you time later! Eye color, hair color, height, full name, nickname, age.
5. Make a short list of distinct locations.
6. If you don't have a lot of time to prepare, a setting or plot familiar to you may be easier. If you choose to explore new territory, there's always Youtube videos you can fast forward through.
7. Name any pets and note their breed and descriptions.
8. Create a loose outline, hitting the 10K points of your story (see Chapter 7, "Using an Outline") At the very minimum, brainstorm the opening, key points, and ending of your story.

That's it. Ready or not, let's go! You can do this!

9

USING AN OUTLINE

There are two approaches to writing a 50K word novel. The first, outlining, can give you a great chance of success, so you don't write yourself into a corner, for example. The second, pantsing or writing it by the seat of your pants, could be nerve-wracking but can result in a more dynamic, fun story.

I usually have good intentions to outline a book. I either outline it to every detail, and then have to revise my story later because my characters, like robots, did exactly what I wanted them to do. Or, I start out with an outline, and stop following it early on. Because any character that lives and breathes in your imagination is a troublemaker and thumbs their noses at the author, the ingrates.

So here's my thoughts on using an outline as it relates to getting word counts this fast. It works great for some people. If you like to outline your books, good for you. Your story will most likely chug along nicely.

Don't worry about an outline killing that adventuresome writing spirit as you draft your 50K words. Its usefulness lies in giving you confidence that if all else fails, you have an exit strategy.

You do not have to follow an outline to a T. If your creative mind deviates from your plot, let it. There are no rules. You need to get from 0 to 50K and if it means you need to have your heiress do something that has firefighters coming to her rescue and it wasn't in the outline, do it!

If you're a pantser like me, don't despair. 50,000 divides neatly into 5 10Ks. Know your beginning and ending (to the best of your ability). Then, at each 10,000 point (which you plan to come to at the end of each day with this experiment), what is happening in the story?

Here's the simple outline I used for *Billionaire Bunker*.

10K Blaze survives an explosion but is chased by assassin. Cin is kidnapped.

20K Blaze finds Cin, who hates his guts for compromising the safety of her grandfather.

30K Blaze and Cin deny their attraction while fighting off setbacks and zombies.

40K Blaze gets in a big pickle and takes Cin to his bunker to find a solution.

50K Stupendous ending with an HEA (Happy Ever After)

The nice thing with the 10K point is it acts as mile markers on this marathon journey. Each 10K notch will help motivate you for the next one. You can also use them as checkpoints to ensure your plot is going along as planned.

Sometimes I get organized enough to plan out scenes. I have a rough idea of the scene and write prompts like "Go to Burano." Or, "Proposal scene."

What if you want to write your story beyond 50K? That is fine. Just plan it out by the next 10K, and so on. Some genres, especially fantasy, lend themselves well to longer word counts.

I would caution you against planning a longer book for this project, however. For one, you can type The End and then go back and add words to flesh out your story. Another thing to consider is, how motivated do you think will you be finishing past 50K once your deadline is over?

~

Divide your story into smaller turkeys

One year, I went to the store and bought two 13-lb turkeys because they were out of 24-lb ones. As much as I wanted to have just one turkey to carve for the sake of presentation, two really makes sense.

(Bear with me for a minute.) Did you know that the larger turkeys are toms and the smaller ones are hens, and typically the hens are more tender? Also, the butcher lady said the larger turkeys take a lot longer to cook and tend to dry out. So it was fortuitous (ha, what a word) that I couldn't find a big one.

How does this relate to writing your novel? If you think of your novel as one 50K turkey, you might get overwhelmed. Instead, divide it up into smaller turkeys.

Since 50K divides nicely into 10,000 portions, think of each section as Set-up, First Major Conflict, Build-up, Second Major Conflict, and Resolution. I made those up, in case you were wondering. I know there are lots of other story beat methods out there, but I like to keep them simple in my mind.

Challenge: Break your story into fifths.

Set-up: What is the story problem? Who are the major players? Why should the reader care?

First Major Conflict: Small conflicts lead up to a big one. Not impossible to overcome, but pretty serious.

Build-up: There's a lot going on in this section. There's also a bit of slice of life scenes that might not be exciting but are important to the advancement of the plot. The main characters are working toward their goals, together or against each other's.

Second Major Conflict: Lay on the conflict thick here. The romance will be derailed. If it's a thriller, someone dies, potentially. All looks hopeless.

Resolution: The hero or heroine or both will either achieve or fail at their main goal/s.

10

UNDERSTANDING YOUR CHARACTERS

I HAVE LISTED character information below that you can use as you plan your story. If you don't know everything right off, that's fine. As you write your story, note details as they come up. This is also helpful if you are writing series so that bringing back recurring characters would be easy peasy. You can use sheets of paper, or my Series Planner.

Name
Nickname
Age
Birthdate
Eye color
Hair color
Height
Ethnicity
Vehicle Make / Year
Personality
Pet/s

. . .

Characteristics
: Weaknesses:
Strengths / Redeeming qualities:
Goal/s:
Obstacle/s to goal/s:
Past history affecting present day:
Hang-up/s about love / life:
How character changes in the story:

Family
: Birth order
Father
Mother
Siblings

Work / Employment
: Company name
Occupation
Co-workers
Other Details

11

50K IN 5 DAYS SCHEDULE

After I finished my 2022 NaNoWriMo project, several author friends asked me what kind of schedule I kept, and if I got any sleep. The answer to the latter is, yes for the most part, amazingly enough. (I was writing about zombies but I didn't want to be a sleepless zombie!) In writing *Billionaire Bunker*, here was my day to day schedule:

Day 1

    7:00 to 8:00 a.m. – Social media

    8:00 to 9:00 a.m. – Walked dog and chores

    9:00 a.m. to 4:00 p.m. – Finished and revised a different manuscript

    4:00 p.m. – Reviewed my notes for *Billionaire Bunker*

    5:30 to 6:00 — Horse chore

    6:00 to 9:00 — Family time

    9:00 to 10:00 — Psyche myself to start a new novel

    10:00 – 11:50 p.m. – Writing sprints

    Midnight – Went to bed

                            . . .

Day 2
    7:00-8:00 a.m. – Social media
    8:00-9:00 a.m. – Walked dog and chores
    9:00 a.m. to 4:00 p.m. – Writing sprints
    4:00 to 5:30 p.m. – Prepared for City Council and ate dinner
    5:30 p.m. – Horse chore
    6:30 to 9:00 p.m. – City Council
    9:00 to 10:00 p.m. – Walked the dog
    10:00 to 11:50 p.m. – Writing sprints
    Midnight – Went to bed

Day 3
    7:00 to 8:00 a.m. – Social media
    8:00 to 9:30 a.m. - Walked the dog
    9:30 to 5:30 p.m. - Writing sprints
    5:30 to 6:00 p.m. – Horse chore
    6:00 to 9:00 p.m. – Dinner and relaxation
    9:00 to 11:50 p.m. – Writing sprints
    Midnight – Went to bed

Day 4 (Hubby was off and home today)
    7:30 a.m to 11:30 a.m. – Writing sprints
    11:30 a.m. to 12:20 p.m. – Walked dog with hubby
    12:30 p.m. to 7:00 p.m. – Writing sprints
    7:00 to 8:00 p.m. – Dinner
    8:00 to 11:55 p.m. – Writing sprints

Day 5
    12:00 a.m. to 1:38 a.m. – Writing sprints

2:00 a.m. – Went to bed

In summary, with practice and fast typing I was getting 10,000 words between 9-5 and then 2,000 after dinner for three hours. I averaged 650 to 750 words per sprint of 20 on and 10 off. I could have stopped at 10K; An additional 2K at night was icing on the cake.

I went to bed at midnight. Woke about 7. Walked the dog and did chores until 9 or 9:30. Ate a quick lunch between sprints. By 5 p.m. I'd get my 10K. Did horse chore at 5:30. I am usually not this productive without a deadline or goal to work up to. On the last night I wanted to get to 50K so I pushed until 1:30 a.m.

Challenge: What schedule will work for you to get your 50K in 5 Days?

12

WHEN LIFE HAPPENS

ONE YEAR I was doing NaNoWriMo, I had committed to babysitting my grandbaby for two days. It's a fun gig; one that I am grateful I can do due to a time-flexible career. Although I wanted to get some headway with my writing challenge, I didn't expect to get any work done. I wanted to be present for the baby when he was awake.

Luckily, not only did I get to enjoy my grandson, he napped several times in the day so I still had a chance to get down some words. After my radical revision where I pretty much started over, I amassed 2,069 words on babysitting day. Not too shabby.

Writing around real life is tricky; NaNo'ing with such a busy November schedule is super tricky. Here are some things I have done to still continue to produce words.

1. I get to work as early as I can. I walk the dog first thing, shower and then get down to business. I used to shower at the end of the day, but that still means disruption just when I am getting in the groove of my writing.

2. Think about your story throughout the day. Even with lots of family goings-on, there's the commute time, driving around, pushing the baby in the stroller. Think through your plot and scenes so that once you can really write, you already have some ideas.
3. Get in the mood. When I write, I put on the same Pandora radio station. The music cues my brain to transition into my series world right away.
4. Write to the time you have. So you only have an hour. Or a half. Or 15 minutes. Set the timer and write as much as you can toward your story. It's easy to be tempted to not even try because you have to overcome inertia. Do not give in. Stay strong and write.
5. Avoid the *Great British Baking Show* and other distractions. While I was tending the grandbaby, my daughter watched an episode of the GBBS. She offered to leave it on for me. I declined. I know myself; I can easily get sucked into a Netflix show. I have told myself that I can watch a good show *after* I finish my manuscript. Or maybe on Saturday night when I am just chilling with the fam.
6. Prepare meals for the week. Before I tended the grandbaby, I prepped three meals that could be easily heated up. It really helps to maximize productivity when you're not spending that hour before dinner prepping a complex meal. Bonus: you're not just eating ramen or putting a lot of the onus on your spouse or other family members to fix meals.

(Although if they can help with some of the meals, then bonus!)
7. Once I reach my goal, and if I have extra time, I push a bit, and then stop. I am sometimes tempted to work throughout the night, but I consciously don't.
8. Clear your calendar. Whether it's NaNo or just my next manuscript, I avoid appointments. I tell family and friends that I would be available again in a week or two. This helps me stay in the groove of my story and keep chugging along.
9. Write during holiday downtimes. Shop, sleep in, watch Netflix—it is morning after Thanksgiving and you could choose to do any of that. Instead you choose to write. Everyone is sleeping in from too much turkey the night before. Take advantage of the quiet and slay those words.

Challenge: Will you work or take a break during the holidays? Be intentional with this decision so you can still carve out time for your family.

13

WRITING CHARACTERS WITH DEPTH

ONE OF THE keys to writing a novel fast is having well-developed characters. Here are some things to try:

1. Give them secrets. They could be secrets you already know from the outset, or, surprise yourself along with your readers. This will give them an air of mystery and will keep your reader curiosity burning.
2. Let your characters explore their deep dark secrets with a confidante. That will make for a revealing conversation.
3. Trust your characters. If they diverge from the storyline, follow them and record what they say and do. You do not have to keep it for your final draft, but the words will get you closer to 50K and give you insight into a character. I have often done this, unsure if the tangent will be useful. Happily, I usually like the scene well enough I keep it.

4. Have your character interact with their family members in a high-emotion event. Not only will this give you a peek into your characters and their families, but readers absolutely enjoy seeing these relationships at play. You could even try having families who are opposite of each other meet.
5. Have your character visit a different setting and record their reaction and how they are seeing the place for the first time.
6. Keep your reader guessing. Zig and zag with character pivot points in the story. For example, in one of my cowboy romances, an heiress comes to a bed and breakfast penniless and asks for a cleaning job. I could have done the stereotypical rich-girl-can't-clean act but I didn't...and as a result my plot took a more interesting turn.

14

HOW TO UP YOUR WORD COUNT

Having rapid released a 50,000-word novel monthly in recent years, where I usually have to come up with 10K words in a day to meet a deadline, here are some techniques I've found effective.

1. Motivate yourself with a deadline. For *Billionaire Bunker*, I wanted to be done with my 50K words before I spent Day 5 at at my daughter-in-law's baby shower. I got my words by 1:38 a.m. that morning.
2. Sprint with others. I sprint with other authors in a Facebook group 20 minutes on 10 minutes off. I like taking that 10 minute break so that my brain can rest and recharge. Some people take 25 minutes. It's a hard amount of time for me because the rest period ends so fast that I start the next one late. Experiment to see what length of time works for you.

3. If you can't find anyone to sprint with, set your timer anyway. Only drawback to this is, it's easy to slack off.
4. To find other sprinters, do a search on Facebook. One I highly recommend is called Writing Sprints. They do contests and other motivators. I cannot stress enough that accountability and my competitiveness account for my highest word counts.
5. I'm a control freak when it comes to sprinting, I will admit. I like timing because I am relentless. I start at the top of the hour or at :30 and I come back to say stop 20 minutes later. Sprint after sprint, all day long. Sometimes, coming to Facebook sprints with just me, myself, and I, I feel like I am announcing my progress to the void. But I tell myself it doesn't matter as the words keep piling up.
6. Between sprints, I take care of phone calls, design ads, interact on social media, run laundry, and do other in-house errands. Some things really do take under 10 minutes.
7. When you are sprinting, stick to sprinting. Check your social media between sprints. Let your calls go to voicemail. Tell your family to talk to you between sprints.
8. Stretch and stand often. I danced between sprints.
9. Keep your fingers constantly moving. I typically average 400-500 words per 20 minute sprints. I was getting 750 to 900 words this way.

10. Stand at your kitchen counter and lean into your keyboard. Pound away like your life depends on it.
11. Eliminate distractions. I took care of must-do chores before I started and did not worry about anything else until I got my words for the day. My family is on notice I am sprinting, which means I can talk to them between rounds.
12. Play music that inspires you. I played bold, energetic instrumental music (Lindsey Stirling) and my fingers typed to the faster beat. The music matched what I was writing—suspense.
13. If I add an important plot detail that will affect earlier text I make a note to add it later. I don't go back to fix things.
14. Improve your personal record. Get more words the next sprint, or the next day. A few books ago, I was talking with a fellow sprinter who said she gets over 900 words in 20 minutes, so I thought I would aim for that at least. When I got past 900, I thought, why not aim for at least 1000? I managed to get it.
15. Avoid the backspace key. Even if I mess up I hit the backspace sparingly, telling myself I could catch it all later on spell check. Just typed, typed, typed.
16. I clear my mind of worries. I write down to-do lists in my planner, and schedule them for days when I am not sprinting. I keep my Saturdays free for catch-up.
17. Keep typing...even if you have to make things up or the plot isn't making sense. Keep typing.

Hopefully the momentum will smooth things out.
18. If a chapter is giving you fits, mark it in the document with ##, skip it, and then go back to it.
19. Take your time to savor and enjoy scenes. Describe what the characters are experiencing in detail. (But don't make it so you are boring the reader to tears with mundane details.)
20. Pick a scene where you mostly tell, and write out what happened in detail. Add a dream sequence that could give the reader insight into your characters biggest fears.

Challenge: What is your word count personal record? Try different length sprints and record your results. Increase your word count each time until the speed becomes natural. Keep pushing . . . you are only limited by what you believe. If you have lower counts, it's okay. Improve on the next ones.

15

RECORDING YOUR WORD COUNT

One of the biggest game-changers for me in my quest to write faster was to record my word counts. By doing so, I could figure out the average speed it takes me to get a certain number of words, and how long it took me to write a certain novel. It is a satisfying visual record of milestones in your journey to finishing your book. I know of authors who swear by digital apps or computer spreadsheets.

I like to record mine on paper, which is why I created my *Series Planner*. Here is one way you could track your word count:

Date | Time | Start Count | End Count | Words Written

P.S. Get my free, downloadable *50K to 5 Days Novel Planner*, which includes a word count tracker, at www.jewelallen.com/get-a-free-book

16

SELF-CARE

WRITING FAST CAN BE PUNISHING for your body. You wouldn't think that something as sedentary as writing could be unhealthy, but it can be, if you're not careful. I know of a lot of authors who have wrist and back injuries, among other health issues, related to writing for long periods at a time.

How to survive 10K-word days:

1. Use an ergonomic keyboard. I got a cheap one from Amazon that plugs into my laptop's USB port. It was partly so I can write fast and also because I have worn out my laptop keys over the years and they are on the fritz.
2. Stretch and stand often. I danced at my desk between sprints. Sometimes during sprints.
3. Get some sleep. I produce better words when I am alert. Since I track my words by the day, I end at midnight and get up at 6 or 7.
4. I write either at my bar-height office desk or our bar-height kitchen island. Typing while

standing helps with the angle of my elbows which avoids wrist strain.
5. Get fresh air. Take the dog for a walk. While on these walks I oftentimes come up with solutions to a plot hole by the time I get back.

Challenge: Identify changes in your life you need to do to practice more self-care.

- _____
- _____
- _____
- _____
- _____
- _____

17

REST AND RECHARGE

I REMEMBER those first few NaNo's I participated in. I divided 50,000 words by 30 days and aimed to write that much each day: 1,667 words. Some days I wrote more than others, but often I fell short and had to make it up. When I did good, I marked that day on a calendar with a sticker.

As I've been able to increase my daily output by sprinting with other authors, more consistently to 10K a day, I've allowed myself breaks. I don't write on Sundays. Saturdays get so busy with family events, I don't count on that day being highly-productive.

Although it's very tempting to write constantly, try to rest and recharge between writing bouts. Instead of staying up, get some sleep. Even though the word count matters, having quality output will save you revision time later.

One year along with NaNo, I was in the throes of preparing my daughter's upcoming wedding. I had been putting off making her invitation, as I told my hubby, "because of NaNo." He said, "NaNo can wait."

I might have taken offense in the past, but it was a good

reminder to me of what's truly important. I made the invitation on Canva *and* still got some words.

My husband has come to accept that, every November, I burrow into my writing hole and rarely emerge. But in the middle of one writing project, I went with him to look at a car and on impulse invited him to try a new restaurant for lunch. It was fun, and gave me some much needed balance.

List things you can do to rest and recharge:

- _____
- _____
- _____
- _____
- _____
- _____

18

START YOUR STORY

THE DAY IS HERE and you are feeling unprepared. You had good intentions to have your story outlined and mapped out on your calendar, but life happened and so here we are. No plan in the horizon but with ambitious word count goals.

If you already have your novel outlined and prepped, great job! You can skip this part. But if not, read on...

It's not too late to prepare to write 50,000 words. Not just words either, but good ones. So that when you're done with your 50K, you don't have to spend a ton of time making sense of your story.

I am a huge proponent of sprinting with other writers, especially during your 50K-word challenge. Everyone is churning out words and keeping each other accountable. The energy is infectious. Work that to your advantage.

Find a supportive writing sprint group to join. For me, the FB group Writing Sprints has been consistently great. Sprint for one or two 20-minute intervals and write down an outline. No writing sprint group? Set a timer and sprint against yourself. The key is to not overthink this exercise.

Just sprint-write the barebones plot of your story. Get

into the heads of your characters and write the plot points from their perspective. Start capturing their personality.

Letting your mind explore all sorts of possibilities makes for a richer, exciting, and fun writing experience. Get your story mapped out, take your writing vehicle out on the road and enjoy the unplanned diversions along the way.

Challenge: Brainstorm openers you can use to hook your reader into your story.

- _____
- _____
- _____
- _____

19

HOW TO FIX A SUCKY OPENING (WITHOUT TRASHING THE WHOLE THING)

When the kids were younger, and they were enthralled by certain books, I would ask to look at the book they were reading, specifically at the opening paragraph to see what makes it hooky.

I had every intention of noting what makes an opening hooky, but I didn't. (Missed opportunity.) Suffice to say that unless the author was lucky to nail it from the get-go, that hooky opening most likely was the result of good editing.

You don't have the same luxury to look upon your NaNoWriMo project and tweak it to perfection. There isn't time. Also, if you do, it will most likely derail your progress.

I didn't follow my own advice in 2021. After the first day of NaNo, I was up to 1,770 words. Day 2 and I was back to 800.

Since then, I normally don't rewrite, let alone delete words. Typically, even if I mess up, I keep writing. My NaNo mantra is, I can always fix that later.

But the one in 2021 started off all wrong. And the new opening felt so right. From there, I didn't change things drastically.

That is one way.

The other way is to keep writing forward. Avoid looking back at the opening, or you will nitpick it. Make a note of what needs to be changed in that earlier section and write according to that change moving forward.

That said, you should at least nail the following from the get-go:

1. How do you want to make the reader feel? Set the mood. Is your story serious? Funny? Sassy? Reflective?
2. A general feel for the characters. Oftentimes, I don't know them completely until they walk onto the stage. But in general, it helps to peg their personality type. Before my rewrite, my characters seemed like cardboard figures. After, I pegged the hero as "calm" and the heroine as "intense."
3. What point-of-view is best for the story? Experiment with a paragraph or two and pick one. Same with the tense--past or present.

20

MAKING YOUR STORY FLOW

Just because you are writing fast does not mean you have to write a pedestrian novel. I don't like time-consuming revisions so I try to nail what I want this first time through. If I struggle, I write plainly or indicate with a placeholder, ##, that I need to find a better word or research a detail.

The most amazing feeling is writing in a dream state, when the words flow. Here are some things I have done to help this along:

1. Put in scenes that are inherently exciting. Brainstorm with someone to get ideas.
2. Add humor, emotion or setting, or a combination of the three.
3. Bring together two characters with opposing goals. Invariably, they will breathe life into your manuscript which means it will be more engaging to write--and read.
4. Add lively dialogue with banter, confrontation, or secret emotions that a reader could sense between the lines.

5. Discover your character's backstory through internal monologue or dialogue if the story allows for it. Don't be so over-indulgent that you slow down the story so much or for too long.
6. Write to your strengths. I don't write just romance, I usually have an element of suspense. I also grew up in the Philippines. I incorporated all this *Billionaire Bunker*, which made my storyline more unique and natural to my storytelling style.
7. Have the characters talk to, or interact, with each other. It's not only great for word count, but it also gives you insight into your characters. Even if you salvaged only a portion of this, hopefully your characterization will be stronger.
8. When you are writing a scene, really delve into the emotion behind each action, and then wring out some more. When you feel, you make the reader feel.
9. Let your character have a bad day. Let them throw a tantrum or act out. In other words, let them be human. This will enrich your characterization.
10. Alternate your pacing between moody scenes making the setting come alive for the reader, and fast-paced action or dialogue.

Challenge: What things would you like to try to make your story flow better?

- _____
- _____
- _____
- _____
- _____

21

MAKING YOUR WORDS COUNT

THE FIRST BOOK I SELF-PUBLISHED, *Ghost Moon Night*, ran 80,000 words and took a lot of revisions. It was a paranormal mystery with tons of world-building. I about wanted to give up several times were it not for the encouragement of my author friend. 50-some odd books later, I am able to write a cleaner draft to meet a rapid release schedule.

It takes 50,000 words to win a writing challenge like NaNoWriMo. Wouldn't it be nice to keep most of the words that you started with once you are in the revision process? You might as well make all those words count.

P.S. I am not advocating for perfection. Especially since it might lead to paralysis. (Keep typing!)

Here's how to make your words count:

1. Make each scene contribute to your story arc.
2. Let the action in your chapters propel your plot forward.
3. Have your characters act consistent with their personality.

4. Ensure there is conflict until the end to keep the reader engaged. If it's boring, you need to throw in more conflict.
5. Give your characters and conflict depth. Mine your deep-seated fears, dreams, and experiences and channel them into your story.
6. If you are writing a mystery, don't worry about setting up clues or motivation or figuring out all the red herrings right off. I usually go back through my document and plant them subtly throughout the earlier text.

22

K-DRAMA YOUR WAY TO A FABULOUS NOVEL

It was movie night in November 2021, and the hubby and I settled in to browse Netflix movies. Guess what series was trending to the top Netflix spot that weekend? Nope, it wasn't *Squid Game*, but close. It was *Hellbound*, another Korean series, based on a Webtoon. This time, *Hellbound* took 24 hours to reach the number one spot. (SG took 4 days.)

If you haven't watched any Korean movies yet, it's time to pay attention. Because Korean filmmakers know a thing or two about pulling an audience along.

For me, my initiation began with *Crash Landing on You*. By the time I started, all episodes were out, so I binged all 16 episodes in one weekend. I loved it. CLOY was a cinematic experience I have never had before.

So what do Korean filmmakers do that we can apply to novel-writing?

1. Put your characters in constant peril.
2. Create unforgettable side characters—yes, even the walk-on.

3. Add humor in unexpected places. It is a great release of tension (especially with peril). And then get back to business.
4. Start with a jaw-dropping story question and keep your audience guessing until the end.
5. Put your characters in tough situations and force them to grow. Make them choose between two equally important things.
6. Make your characters struggle over relatable, universal themes: belonging, freedom from debt, fear of death and damnation.

Think of your characters and brainstorm what funny and tough situations you can put them through:

- _____
- _____
- _____
- _____
- _____
- _____

23

HOW TO FIX A FRANKEN-PLOT

As you go along drafting your novel, you might decide to take it a different trajectory than you had planned. Which means a domino effect--your entire plot will have to be changed earlier in the draft.

All is not lost.

Write on like you had planned this all along, while making a note in caps somewhere of a plot change at this spot. This is also a good time to note what changes you would need to do in revision. Doesn't have to be complex ideas, just even a word or two.

And then write on as though the change were in place from the get-go. Do not worry about fixing the rest of the story at this point, or you'll be tempted to erase words (not good for a word count challenge) and possibly create a confusing Frankenstein of mashed up parts.

Later, when you revise, make changes in small amounts. Resist the temptation to overhaul the whole story. Sometimes, all that is needed is a sentence or two of explanation.

But what if the change you've applied relates to someone's personality or character? For example, in one of my novels, I started out with a nice heiress, then decided to make her spoiled. I still went ahead and kept drafting forward. I just had to make sure she was consistent in the earlier portion of the story with the change.

In the back of your mind, you will most likely worry that your story will be one hot mess by the time you finish it. Keep powering to the end and you just might be pleasantly surprised that your Franken-novel actually isn't as bad as you think.

Or at least, not as hopeless.

24

SHORING UP THE MIDDLE SAG

At several points during your manuscript, you will absolutely hate your story. You will think it is worthless, cheerless, and all sorts of -less, and why are you even trying to write a book? And 50K words even!

For me, this usually happens at the 15 to 20K point, when I'm feeling tapped out of all my clever plot points and look beyond to the 50K finish line as though it's a mirage in the desert.

It seems the middle is where I throw in everything but the kitchen sink (true story: my husband was a church missionary in Korea and once saw a man carrying a big bundle to the bus stop including a kitchen sink). Just to add the words.

Which isn't altogether a bad plan. Sometimes, it helps to pursue a conversation between characters to uncover motivation. However, where it is unwieldy is adding stuff that is not relevant to the plot. It could certainly add words, but they will most likely end up junked later. All that effort, ugh.

Here are some ways to combat the Middle Sag.

1. Introduce an eccentric character or plot twist.
2. Write in the point of view of a secondary character. You might or might not keep this chapter, but it might inspire you about a character or your story. I did this once with a cowboy story, wrote from the POV of a horse ... and kept it. My beta reader was pleasantly surprised and loved it.
3. Be sure to add conflict whenever you can. When my manuscript lags and I am like, "This scene is boring and is begging to end," I usually discover that everyone is acting too nice. (True story: when I first met my husband I thought he was too "nice" and clean-cut. I wasn't too interested in him. A few months, scruff, and longer hair later, I agreed to go on a date with him. So it works for relationships too!)
4. If a character is expected to do A, make him/her do B. Try to keep the action consistent with their character.
5. Get your characters in trouble and *let them figure out how to get out of it*. The second part is important. Your characters aren't helpless. They are smart and will figure things out even better than you, the author. Let them pleasantly surprise you.
6. Bored with a scene? Abort and go on to a scene you're excited about. Once you are reenergized about your story, go back to the problem spot, or maybe it's a good indication the scene wasn't necessary to begin with.

Midway through your novel, you should be building up

to a crisis point where the characters will have to act if they really want to reach their goals. (Ideally, they do, or you won't have much of a story.) What that means is that you will make life difficult for them. If it looks like they will kiss, drop a distraction. If it looks like they are playing nice, let them get unruly. It's not only essential for your character to work towards their goals, it is absolutely crucial, if you want to keep going another 25K words.

Remember, you only have to keep this up in this middle sections. The next one, you will make things worse and maybe even make it seem like they will all crash and burn.

And you can lean against that post, nod and feel all-powerful.

25

STICK TO IT

ONCE AGAIN, about two-thirds into your manuscript, you will be staring down a very big realization about your NaNoWriMo project: it is one big mess. You are simply sure of this. Which might or might not be true. You might even be tempted to go back and edit it, to shore up your losses.

Do not do it.

From here on, you must move forward with your manuscript even though you think it might not be worth saving. Especially if you have a massive amount of words already.

True story: In 2018, I wrote a Christmas romance that I was sure was worthless. About halfway through, I was so bored with my story, I introduced an out-there sub-plot and characters, which I thought derailed the whole book. I wanted to scrap my story so badly.

After I won NaNoWriMo that year, I didn't even bother to read the story. I shelved it for a whole year, until the following October, when, out of curiosity, I dug it up. I started reading it. It wasn't perfect, but it was pretty good. Three years later, *A Cowboy for Christmas* has been one of my best sellers and has been a great reader lead-in into my Riverdale Ranch Romance Series.

26

FINISH STRONG

I USED to be a ghostwriter of memoirs. Clients came to me with a similar story, over and over. They had started their book, but didn't know how to get past that first or first few chapters. Some had a document of memories but didn't know how to mold it into a readable story.

In essence, people hired me to help them finish what they started. I got really good at that—finishing a book, with all its imperfections. There would be room for revision later.

The key to finishing? It's having a goal and finally saying the book is done.

If you are down to the wire, if you have one more day left before your deadline, or if you haven't reached your word count goal, this is the time to summon up that last push.

Finish what you started.

Some finishing tricks that have worked for me:

1. Towards the end of my story, when the end is in sight and I want to write faster, I open up a different file for each sprint and write a scene to

the end in that 20 minute sprint. I watch the word counter in the bottom left corner and aim to cross 1k each time.
2. Take stock of where you are at in your story. Is it time to wrap things up or do you still need to add more words? It is like Christmas tree trimming. You have a beautiful tree you started with, which you can add ornaments to. Simple or elaborate, it is up to you!
3. If you write The End before you get 50K, don't worry. For *Billionaire Bunker*, I still needed 5K words, so I added a Christmas day scene, a prologue, an epilogue, and a wedding scene. By the time I was done, I was 116 words over 50K.

27

AFTER THE 50K

You have a 50K-word manuscript. Congratulations! After you pat yourself on the back and do a celebratory dance, I suggest you do the following:

1. Take a well-deserved break. Take the day off. Watch a movie just for fun. Eat out with your loved ones. Let your brain heal and rest. But not for too long. You will need to be back to your manuscript if you want to self-publish it soon.
2. Now's the time to share your accomplishment to get your potential readership engaged and excited.
3. If you need to add more words to your novel, do so and finish it. Repeat step 1.
4. Pick a day when you have a stretch of time and open your manuscript. It's okay to be scared. I always have to open one eye first, before the other. Take a deep breath and read it in one sitting, if possible. Read it like a potential reader. Don't be too hard on yourself. It's

probably not as bad as you think. Fix typos as you go along. Make notes on a sheet of paper or in the margins of big picture things that you need to fix.
5. Note the timeline and adjust accordingly. This is how I check mine: as I read the manuscript, I draw up the timeline and write what happens on Day 1, etc., making sure the timeline is believable.
6. Fix any spots where you've marked with your placeholder. Substitute the right words. Fact check. Name your characters.
7. Re-read the manuscript again. This time, make the changes. I edit sprint with other authors, too, so that I could revise my book faster.
8. Don't change anything in major way. Drastic changes require drastic changes throughout your manuscript. Maybe your manuscript is that bad, but I doubt it. A sentence or two usually can help fix or explain plot holes. I think about this whenever I am backing a boat trailer. If I yank every which way, my trailer trajectory goes haywire; keep calm and my backing goes pretty smooth.
9. Chillax. We are our biggest critics. Sometimes, the things I worry about in my manuscript are never mentioned by my readers. Don't sweat the small details.
10. Arrange one or more beta readers. Beta readers have a special place in author heaven. I hire a professional beta reader who reads my book within a week and gives me overall feedback. It is best to pick a beta reader who reads and/or

writes in your genre. You can connect with other authors on Facebook as I have, or ask readers in your social circle, for referrals.

11. Stick to your guns. If you have been inspired to try a unique opener or treatment to this story, leave it in. See what your beta reader thinks. If they hate it, maybe reconsider.
12. When you get the feedback from your beta reader, eat chocolate and then dig in. Again, don't make drastic changes. Have I said that before?
13. Hire a developmental editor. If you are fairly new to self-publishing and/or writing, you will benefit from this step. I did this early on in my publishing career. My editors (I used several, alternating, especially during my rapid releases, so I don't burn them out) taught me a lot about writing and editing, techniques that I apply subconsciously now.
14. Make the changes.
15. Hire a proofreader who will catch your typos.
16. Run a spell-check.
17. Run a grammar-check.
18. Put out a call for Advance Review Copy (ARC) readers and request them to let you know if they see any other typos.
19. Make suggested changes, if any.
20. Hit publish!

28

PARTING THOUGHTS

Our family has had a yearly Thanksgiving tradition for several years now. We all participate in a Turkey Trot which is not only great exercise and bonding activity, but benefits the food bank (we donate canned goods for our entry).

The past few years, I have walked because running is too hard on my knees (not to mention I feel like I'm going to die). Last year, I brought my 7-month-old puppy Lily.

I could have been down on myself for not running and clocking in a great time like others who are more fit or are faster, but I am just grateful that I can move my body, my puppy is nice to people and other animals, and that I finished the race.

In publishing, us authors tend to compare ourselves to others who are faster, make more money, or are more popular. It's a natural tendency. Society (especially social media) likes to measure and reward those who are higher-ranked, have more fans, or have more quantifiable success.

They don't see how much of a win it is for some of us to

be brave and write a page or two towards our dream of a story. Or how each book makes us a stronger writer.

Regardless of whether or not you can write 50,000 words in 5 days, what truly matters is that you are moving in the right direction and are improving every time.

Best of luck on your writing journey! If you want to join a supportive group of authors wanting to write and publish faster while still striving for balance, join my group on Facebook, Rapid Releasers. Connect with me at www.JewelAllen.com.

∼

Thanks for reading *Rapid Novel*. I hope you've enjoyed it and find it useful. Could you please take a few minutes to leave a review? Thank you! Get my free, downloadable *50K to 5 Days Novel Planner* at www.jewelallen.com/get-a-free-book

29

BONUS: WORD COUNT TRACKER

WORD COUNT TRACKER

BOOK

DATE/TIME	START COUNT	END COUNT	TOTAL

WORD COUNT TRACKER

BOOK

DATE/TIME	START COUNT	END COUNT	TOTAL

WORD COUNT TRACKER

BOOK

DATE/TIME	START COUNT	END COUNT	TOTAL

WORD COUNT TRACKER

BOOK

DATE/TIME	START COUNT	END COUNT	TOTAL

WORD COUNT TRACKER

BOOK

DATE/TIME	START COUNT	END COUNT	TOTAL

WORD COUNT TRACKER

BOOK

DATE/TIME	START COUNT	END COUNT	TOTAL

WORD COUNT TRACKER

BOOK

DATE/TIME	START COUNT	END COUNT	TOTAL

WORD COUNT TRACKER

BOOK

DATE/TIME	START COUNT	END COUNT	TOTAL

WORD COUNT TRACKER

BOOK

DATE/TIME	START COUNT	END COUNT	TOTAL

WORD COUNT TRACKER

BOOK

DATE/TIME	START COUNT	END COUNT	TOTAL

Printed in Great Britain
by Amazon

Printed in Great Britain
by Amazon

Samuele Cortese, E. K.-C. (2006). Sleep and alertness in children with attention-deficit/hyperactivity disorder: a systematic review of the literature. *Sleep, 29*(4), 504-511.

K. Lindstrom, F. L. (2011). Preterm Birth and Attention-Deficit/Hyperactivity Disorder in Schoolchildren. *Pediatrics, 127*(5), 858-865.

Mats Johnson, S. Ö. (2009). Omega-3/Omega-6 Fatty Acids for Attention Deficit Hyperactivity Disorder. *Journal of Attention Disorders, 12*(5).

Megan R. McDougall, D. A. (2006). Having a Co-Twin With Attention-Deficit Hyperactivity Disorder. *Twin Research and Human Genetics, 9*(1), 148-154.

Natali Golan, E. S. (2004). Sleep disorders and daytime sleepiness in children with attention-deficit/hyperactive disorder. *Sleep, 27*(2), 261-266.

Nigel M. Williams, I. Z. (2010). Rare chromosomal deletions and duplications in attention-deficit hyperactivity disorder: a genome-wide analysis. *The Lancet, 376*(9750), 1401-1408.

Philip Shaw, M. G. (2007). Polymorphisms of the Dopamine D4 Receptor, Clinical Outcome, and Cortical Structure in Attention-Deficit/Hyperactivity Disorder. *Archives of General Psychiatry, 64*(8), 921.

Rosalind J. Neuman, E. L.-W. (2007). Prenatal Smoking Exposure and Dopaminergic Genotypes Interact to Cause a Severe ADHD Subtype. *Biological Psychiatry, 61*(12), 1320-1328.

Ruff, M. E. (2005). Attention Deficit Disorder and Stimulant Use: An Epidemic of Modernity. *Clinical Pediatrics, 44*(7), 557-563.

References

Ajay Singh, C. J. (2015). Overview of attention deficit hyperactivity disorder in young children. *Health Psychology Research, 3*(2).

Amelia Villagomez, U. R. (2014). Iron, Magnesium, Vitamin D, and Zinc Deficiencies in Children Presenting with Symptoms of Attention-Deficit/Hyperactivity Disorder. *Children, 1*(3), 261-279.

Avi Sadeh, L. P.-H. (2006). Sleep in children with attention-deficit hyperactivity disorder: a meta-analysis of polysomnographic studies. *Sleep medicine reviews, 10*(6), 381-398.

Elizabeth Anderson, G. S. (2013). Effects of Exercise and Physical Activity on Anxiety. *Frontiers in Psychiatry, 4.*

Eric Konofal, M. L.-C. (2004). Iron Deficiency in Children With Attention-Deficit/Hyperactivity Disorder. *Archives of Pediatrics & Adolescent Medicine, 158*(12), 1113.

Genevieve Young, J. C. (2005). Omega-3 fatty acids and neuropsychiatric disorders. *Reproduction Nutrition Development, 45*(1), 1-28.

Hechtman, L. (2008). Treatment of adults with attention-deficit/hyperactivity disorder. *Neuropsychiatric Disease and Treatment*, 389.

Joel T. Nigg, A. L. (2015). Variation in an Iron Metabolism Gene Moderates the Association Between Blood Lead Levels and Attention-Deficit/Hyperactivity Disorder in Children. *Psychological Science, 27*(2), 257-269.

helps with ADHD symptoms, and I have included plenty of ways in this book in which you can do. Understand that your brain is biologically different from that of others and so you react differently to situations. After a certain point of time, ADHD patients get accustomed to the constant criticism hurled at them. But it would help if you stood up for yourself because you have done nothing wrong. And while you do that, celebrate all the small victories down the road. Every little success counts because you are putting in a lot of effort, and you deserve to be appreciated. I want to end this book by saying that you should find your own tribe and connect with more people who have ADHD through the various support groups. Connecting with others who have the same problem will not only make you feel understood but also appreciated.

Finally, I would be grateful if you left a review on Amazon if this book was able to provide you with the information you were looking for!

not only help you uncover your strengths but also show you that you are good at so many things.

People with ADHD have a hard time saying no. Even after you have followed all the strategies mentioned in this book, you will struggle if you cannot set boundaries. Don't let the people in your life walk all over you. There has to be a line that you cannot let others cross. Spend time with people who support you and who have the same qualities as you. This will make the process easier. When you are hanging out with people who see the best in you and support you the way you are, you will automatically feel happier.

Having said all this, I would like to remind you that you should take time off every week for yourself. During this time, do all the things that you love to do. This can mean anything – going on a road trip with friends, a backyard barbeque party, or even going to a book club. It is very similar to recharging batteries.

You cannot run away from the fact that your mood is going to change after every few minutes. But you need to come up with better ways to deal with those changes. Don't put the blame on someone else or waste time thinking about why you have mood swings. You need to figure out what you can do to tolerate that moment and spend it doing something that doesn't involve hurting others. You can go and play tennis or have a coffee at your favorite café.

The ADHD brain is wired to dive deep into the all-or-nothing thinking process. Giving structure to your life

It is time that you stop beating yourself up and start taking action towards leading a better life. I know that you must have heard comments like 'loser' and 'incompetent' from your colleagues or friends. But you cannot let these petty comments define you. Stop the negative thinking right now and replace it with positivity. I know that there are a lot of obstacles in your path, but you have to learn to deal with them one by one. If you try to handle them all at once, you will become overwhelmed. At the same time, you need to take your medication on time because the medications, together with therapy, is what will give you dramatic improvement.

Don't judge yourself too harshly – it is never healthy. The emotional pain can get too much, but you simply have to find ways to deal with it. I hope the strategies mentioned in this book help you get through some of the toughest moments. It is easy to beat yourself up, but it is not easy to forgive and move on. With ADHD, it is natural for you to feel self-critical at all times. The root of this problem lies in childhood because that's when ADHD kids are looked upon with displeasure from their teachers and parents. ADHD kids work day and night to get the approval of others, but it is never enough. But now that you are an adult, you need to break free of that cycle, and the strategies mentioned in this book are going to help you a lot.

Stop spending time thinking about your weaknesses because now, you need to focus on your strengths. Make yourself feel good. Take a notepad and make a list of all those things that you are good at. This will

Conclusion

Thank you for reading *Thriving With ADHD Workbook: Guide to Stop Losing Focus, Impulse Control and Disorganization Through a Mind Process for a New Life.* I sincerely hope that this book was able to give you the tools you were looking for, and you were able to clarify your doubts.

Now you have to take your baby steps towards working out all the problems you are facing at living your life with ADHD. So far, we have covered the major aspects of everyone's life and the most common problems that ADHD patients deal with. I want to close with a simple note that sometimes, along your journey, there will come the point when you need to seek help from others. And there is no need to shy away from that. We all need to seek help once in a while, and that is completely okay. That doesn't make you small or inferior. It only makes you stronger.

The symptoms of ADHD can easily overwhelm you and weight you down. If you don't deal with them, they will keep haunting you and hampering your life. By now, you must have understood that the functioning of an ADHD brain is quite different from others. There are different processes that lead to different behaviors. The great impact of these symptoms on a person's emotions is what poses as the major struggle.

At the beginning of this chapter, I told you that you need to know about your triggers. Similarly, you also need to learn about what calms you down. Everyone has a different strategy that works for them, and you need to find yours. If listening to music calms you down, then be it. If a walk around the block to take in the fresh air is what you need, do it. It is like your anger first aid kit, and you need to know your tools.

But to get started with anger management, you need to acknowledge to yourself that you are having a hard time controlling your anger. If nothing works, you should talk to your doctor about it.

Learn to Express Yourself in Other Ways

There are a lot of ways to let your anger out than yelling, shouting, or creating a scene. For this, you have to acknowledge that anger is nothing but an emotion, and it is sending a signal to you that something is really bothering you. When you do that, you will be able to articulate yourself in a better way and, thus, express yourself without hurting someone. It would help if you simply made others hear you, and for that, an angry outburst is not a solution. You need to able to have a proper conversation. For this, you can learn to use the right words. An anger outburst is ingrained in us from a young age because when we are young, anger is how we express our feelings for which we don't have words. But when we grow up, we do have the words, and yet we turn to anger. You have to replace anger as your coping mechanism with something that won't hurt others and also take your pain away.

If you are too angry to talk to someone, then it is better that you don't talk to them at that moment. Reschedule your meeting and speak with them some other time when you are not angry. It will help you analyze their point of view without jumping to any conclusion.

But if you are indeed in an unbearable situation, then you need to take a step back and think about the worst outcome. Well, the worst result might not even occur, but you should always be ready with a plan in case it does. Moreover, like you already know, regulation of emotions is something ADHD patients face a lot of trouble with. So, this exercise can be beneficial to them.

Always Remain Positive

We are now going to discuss an essential step. Staying positive is crucial to deal with all problems in your life. You are bound to come across situations in your life where people will push the buttons, and your anger will cross the threshold. But how you choose to act in that situation is what is most important. When faced with failures, ADHD patients end up overreacting most of the time. That is why having a plan for every situation is important. You also need to have a Plan B in case Plan A does not work. It will make sure that you do not dwell on your failures and always have a path that will help you move on.

One of the key steps to being positive is to pat yourself on the back and congratulate yourself from time to time. Every time you are successful at reigning in your anger and taking control of the situation, congratulate yourself. You deserve that. Your self-esteem will benefit a lot from this exercise, and gradually, you will notice that your relationship with others is also improving.

accumulating and take the shape of a serious anger outburst later.

Breaks should not be a once in a while things. They should be incorporated into your routine in a regular manner so that you don't forget about them. You need to take a break after every hour of work, after every week, after every month, and also after every year. The duration of each of these breaks will be different. You need to plan something special for yourself once a month and a grand trip once a year. It will help you freshen up your mind and return to work with more energy.

Think About the Consequences

This strategy has seemed to work for a lot of people. One of the most common things that you will notice in people with ADHD is that they are not able to control their anger outbursts. In simpler terms, they do not have restraint. That is why you need to take a pause and then think about what your anger is going to bring you. Is it good? The most probable answer is no. Then, take a moment to think about what is you acted in a better way? What if you changed your response to something positive? You should also try to talk to your coach or your friends and discuss the incident that triggered your anger. It might even lead to some self-revelation. You never know what helps in your growth so that the next time it happens, you can respond in a better way.

not taking care of yourself or not noticing the things you should on a daily basis. This means that you need to sleep well. A good sleeping regimen can do wonders for your mood and also increase your threshold for anger. You also need to eat the right kinds of food. A healthy diet is so essential. Also, if you are on any medication for ADHD or anything else, make sure you don't miss out on them.

When you are taking care of yourself, you are giving your body everything it needs to stay well. Your body can function properly only when it gets what it needs. All of these small steps, when seen together, can reduce your symptoms and also help keep your anger in check.

Take Breaks

The next step for anger management is taking breaks. No matter how many things you have on your to-do list, you have to take breaks in between. You will easily burn out if you don't relax and take some rest. Work is important, but so is rest. If you keep the engine of your running for a long time, it is going to wear out soon. The same thing applies to your body. If you want to function healthily, you have to take breaks in between. This will give your mind time to re-energize and feel better. You need to give your spirit the time to refuel so that your anger outbursts don't happen at the most unfortunate moments. What may seem like a subtle grievance now might keep

Whenever you figure out that something is triggering you, note it down. Since ADHD patients have very low impulse control, triggers can take a completely different form and pose far greater challenges. Some triggers are huge, while some are small and minute things.

Once you have made a list of your triggers, it is time you sit down and sort through them one by one. For each one of them, think as to how you can avoid the triggers, and in case you come face to face with it, think of strategies that will help you to keep your anger in control. For example, if you get triggered every time you are stuck in traffic, then you need to change your commute time. For this, you can talk to your employer. But always have a backup plan for every trigger in case the first plan doesn't work.

In case nothing works, you should call up someone you trust or rely on. Let them know beforehand that you are going to call them. Ask that friend to take your mind off the issue that is causing the anger. But if you can't get hold of anyone at that moment, try counting from one to ten slowly and take deep breaths.

Take Care of Yourself

You must be wondering how this is related to managing anger. Well, it is because anger doesn't come to you overnight. It results from keeping things inside of you for too long. It happens because you are

Chapter 10: ADHD Anger Management Tips

There are quite a handful of reasons why people with ADHD struggle to keep their anger in check. If you are struggling with it as well, then you will find a lot of strategies in this chapter that will help you overcome it in no time. One of the major reasons why anger is such a big issue in ADHD patients is the constant mood swings. At one moment, the person is happy and cheerful, and the next moment, they are feeling unsettles and furious. This makes them act in an impulsive manner. Another reason for such anger outbursts is the accumulation of stress in ADHD patients.

Remember that you are not the only one struggling to bring your anger under control. There are plenty of other people like you who are also trying to keep their anger in check. So, here are some constructive ways in which you can manage your anger.

Know What Makes You Angry

So, the first step to overcoming anger is to understand what is making you angry. In simpler terms, you have to identify your triggers. Anger can be triggered in a variety of situations, and it is not always the same for everyone. When you know the situation in which there is a chance of you getting angry, you can take a break and calm yourself down.

these steps, you will gradually see that you are mastering the art of organization.

but it is also very easy to get lost in them. So, it is my advice to you that you keep your to-do lists short. Your list should have the tasks written in bold and big letters and don't list more than five or six tasks on the list. If there any additional tasks, write them on the back of the index card, and you will do those tasks only if you have time left after completing the major ones. When you see that your list is becoming short and you don't have too many things on the same page, you will automatically feel less frustrated. This will make completing tasks much easier.

Limit Your Distractions

There are too many distractions in our everyday life, but there is a way to fight them. You simply have to take the first step. Organizing your life will become way too difficult if you don't steer clear of all the distractions. When you are working, your focus should be solely on your work. Put your phone in the silent mode, and don't look at it for the next fifteen minutes. You can check your email after that and then return back to work for another fifteen minutes. Free your workspace of any clutter. The more things you have on your desk, the more will be the distractions.

Lastly, I would say that you need to take it one project at a time. Once you have set your priority, focus on completing that before moving on to something else. This will ensure that before you start a new task, all the loose ends have been tied up. If you follow all cap. If you are deciding on which sofa you should buy, set a time cap and then make a resolution that you are going to make your final decision before your time cap is over.

Whenever you are making a decision, I know that there are a lot of factors and, thus, a lot of angles to think from. But you need not think about everything. You have to prioritize and think about only some of the factors which are most important to you. It can be practicality, price, aesthetics, or anything else. The factors should be chosen by their importance. Stick to one factor for your ultimate decision.

Don't Over-Commit

We all have a tendency to overcommit. But you have to hold yourself back from doing so. When people have ADHD, they have a hard time keeping track of everything in their life. So, when you over-commit, you have a lot of things on your plate, and you cannot possibly handle all of them. If you spread yourself too thin, none of the tasks can be completed properly. So, commit to one task at a time and don't take up too much work at a time. You have to prioritize your own mental health over anything else.

Your To-Do Lists Should Not Be Too Long

Making to-do lists is definitely a great way to start the day and keep track of all those things you need to do,

Your schedule should not only be about work. You should keep ample space in your schedule for socializing. Taking care of yourself also means that you need to meet people and go out with them. If you are an avid reader, then join a book club. If you love fitness, join a yoga class. Do what you love but make time for yourself.

Another thing that really helps ADHD patients is joining ADHD support groups. These groups can do wonders to how you see your life. They provide a lot of emotional support on days when you don't feel like doing anything. Everything that you are going through, the group members have gone through as well. So, why not share your experiences? There are a lot of in-person and online groups that you can check out.

Make Decisions Within a Time Limit

Making decisions can be quite overwhelming for an ADHD patient, and the main reason behind this is that they end up being so confused that making a decision seems next to impossible. Some patients can even spend weeks agonizing over the same issue over and over again. However, when analyzed by someone else, those decisions should not take you more than a couple of minutes. If you are going through the same thing, then one of the simplest was to solve it is to set a time limit. When you have a time cap, you know that you have to make a decision by the end of that time

Sort through your credit cards and see what you need and what you don't. The more cards you have, the more you will get confused. So, it is always better to stick only a few cards that will give you more benefits than the others. If companies are bothering you with new card offers, read the terms very carefully and then judge whether you truly need them or your current card is enough to cover everything.

Always have a few hundred dollars in your apartment in someplace safe. This will serve as a backup in case the ATMs are closed, or there is a power outrage. If you keep misplacing your wallet every day before leaving the house, try using a wallet that is colorful. When your wallet is black or brown in color, they tend to mix with other things, and you cannot spot them at once. But when it has a bright color, it becomes easier to spot them.

Prioritize Your Happiness and Health

Most people don't realize how important it is to put their health before everything else. No matter where you are, you should always have some extra ADHD medication at hand. Whenever you are writing things in your planner, make sure you check your medication and note down the date when you need to refill it. In this way, you will never run out of medication. You can even set a reminder alert on your phone to remind you when you need to buy new meds. But the date you are setting for refilling your medication should be at least a week before you run out of meds.

also use an app for it. Then, you can set timely reminders for everything that is on your planner.

Organize Your Finances

The next step to becoming organized is to have a look at your finances and make sure everything is in order. The forgetfulness that comes with ADHD often makes people overlook their finances, and by the time they realize that it needs work, it is too late. If you don't want that to happen to you, I think you should review your finances every quarter. Mark a particular date in your planner or calendar when you want to review all your financial statements and make sure you do those things on that date. This should be a comprehensive review and must include your retirement accounts, all your bank accounts, and your investment accounts.

If you do not use online banking, then it is high time that you do so now. It is going to make your life so much easier. Writing checks and doing all the work manually is such a hassle. But when you do it online, it becomes way easier. If you think about all the monthly bills that you have to pay, then online banking can make it a cakewalk because they can be paid automatically. If you are not so savvy with computers and that is what is pushing you back from online banking, don't worry, it's not that tough. But in any case, you can always ask a family member or a friend for help.

enough time in the day for you to do everything, a planner can sort that out for you. You can now keep every errand, every meeting, and every event scheduled so that you don't forget about it. Make sure you keep some time extra on your hands when you note down the event in your calendar. If the meeting is at 2 pm, note down the time as 1:45 pm, so that you have some extra time to give you a cushion.

Once you start maintaining a planner, you will see how your personal and professional life undergoes a huge change. You are going to become so much more productive and no more putting off things for later. If it is included in your planner, you have to do it now. Whatever task we are talking about, a planner will help you stay ahead of things and keep some extra time for you and your family at the end of the day.

Constantly feeling overwhelmed is something very common with ADHD patients, and this leads to an immense amount of stress. But your schedule can be so much less hectic if only you maintain a planner. Every responsibility will be completed seamlessly. You can also use your planner to keep track of what you are eating and whether or not you are doing some regular exercise.

Another important thing to keep in mind is that even when you are maintaining your planner, you need to keep checking it from time to time to ensure that you are not missing out on anything. Make it a habit to note down all your meetings and appointments in the planner. If you don't want to do it manually, you can away. Even if you need to know something about your device, all you need is the model number, and you will find every information online.

- **Free Samples** – Do you feel good when you get free samples with other products or when you travel? Of course, you do but think about all those times when these free samples just keep accumulating, and we never really use them. So, instead of throwing these samples away, you can donate them to those who really need them.

- **Magazines** – Do you have magazines lying around in every room? If yes, then you need to make a list of magazines that you really love to read, and anything that is not on that list should be recycled. Also, prioritize the magazines to see whether you still want to continue your subscription to all of them.

Set a fixed day every month when you will go through your belongings and throw out things you don't need. After that, your focus should be on buying things that you absolutely need. If you don't buy unnecessary things, you will not have clutter in the first place.

Maintain a Planner

When you have ADHD, you often tend to forget things, and that creates even more chaos in life. But a simple solution to this problem is maintaining a planner. So, if you have been feeling that there is not nearest recycling center. Then, visit the supermarket and buy some reusable grocery bags. Keep about five of them in your car so that whenever you go somewhere, you always have one in the car. You should buy a bunch more to keep in your house. But in case you are at a store, and you don't have your reusable bags with you, you can always ask for paper bags.

- **Extension Cords** – I know that most of us are guilty of keeping worn out extension cords in our home. But ask yourself whether you really need so many of them. You can just keep one from each type of cord and throw away the rest.
- **Old Electronics** – Do you hold on to your old gadget even when you have bought a new one? That is how you are giving rise to clutter. You need to get rid of the old one. Or, you can also replace your old one and get a new gadget – this might even save you some money.
- **Extra Bedsheets** – Open your linen closet and see how many bedsheets you have. Every one of us keeps extra bedsheets in case we need them when guests are over. But do you have too many? If so, then you need to discard some of them.
- **Manuals** – In today's when you have everything you need online, why keep accumulating manuals? The first page of the manual might have the warranty card – you can tear it off and throw the rest of the manual

Chapter 9: Tips to Make Your Life More Organized

One of the biggest challenges when a person has ADHD, is to become organized. But it is not something impossible. You can bring structure and discipline to your life if you put in the effort. Always remember that the secret to becoming organized is to follow some simple steps that you can continue doing and having a system that works well for your routine. In this chapter, we are going to have a lot at some simple tips that will help you make your life more organized.

Throw Out What You Don't Need

We all have things in our lives that we keep on accumulating even though we don't need them. And in the case of people with ADHD, these things are even more because they have very poor organizational skills. The more physical clutter you have in your life, the more will be your mental clutter. So, it would be best if you eliminated all those things you don't need from time to time. If you can't figure out where to start, then here are some things that you can throw away –

- **Plastic Grocery Bags** – These things tend to get accumulated in our houses very easily. If you are feeling like going green, just take all the plastic bags that are lying around and visit the

- Tuna and salmon and other fatty fish

If you think that food alone cannot provide your body with the required amount of nutrients, then you can also try taking daily supplements. Talk to your doctor about which supplement will be good for you.

Omega-3-Fatty Acids

These compounds are very important for promoting healthy nerve function and also for keeping your brain in good health. A study was conducted in Sweden, and it found that ADHD symptoms were decreased by 50% when omega-3s were consumed daily in the form of fatty, cold-water fish like salmon, tuna, and sardines (Mats Johnson, 2009).

Dr. Sven Ostlund selected a group of children, and these children were in the age group of 8-18. They consumed fish oil every day. A 25% reduction of ADHD symptoms was noticed in these children within a span of 6 months.

There was another study that showed – the process of breakdown of omega-3s is much easier and faster in patients with ADHD than in those who are not diagnosed with this disorder (Genevieve Young, 2005). Greater levels of improvement in terms of cognitive function and mental focus were observed in those ADHD patients whose levels of omega-3s in blood were low. But you also have to remember that consuming omega-3s doesn't mean they can substitute your normal medications.

Some of the common food items that can provide you with omega-3-fatty acids are as follows –

- Flax seeds
- Chia seeds
- Walnuts

- **Iron** – Tofu, kidney beans, beef, and liver
- **Vitamin D** – Fortified foods, beef liver, egg yolks, and fatty fish
- **Vitamin B-6** – Potatoes, peanuts, fish, and eggs

The regulation of dopamine in your brain is controlled b zinc. In fact, zinc might even be responsible for producing methylphenidate. This particular compound is, in turn, responsible for improving the response of the brain towards dopamine. Inattentiveness has been found in patients who had lower levels of this mineral. Similarly, iron is yet another mineral that holds importance in the production of dopamine.

Iron stores in the body are measured through a compound known as ferritin. A study was conducted, and it showed that ferritin levels were in 18% of kids in the control group as compared to the 84% of kids with ADHD (Eric Konofal, 2004). The symptoms of ADHD have been found to become severe when iron stores were low. The cognitive defects increased too.

Magnesium is responsible for inducing a calming effect, and it is also involved in the production of certain neurotransmitters. Thus, the intake of magnesium helps in increasing concentration and attention.

Some of the examples of complex carbohydrates that should be included in your diet are as follows –

- Lentils and beans
- Brown rice
- Pasta and whole-grain bread
- Vegetables
- Fruits

Vitamins & Minerals

Vitamins and minerals are very important for your body, irrespective of whether you have ADHD or not. They help in improving your alertness and also improves attention.

There have been studies that show ADHD is also linked with deficiencies of certain vitamins and minerals (Amelia Villagomez, 2014). But there is no conclusive evidence stating that a deficiency of any minerals or vitamins leads to ADHD. However, it is also true that when people increased their consumption of these vitamins and minerals, they witnessed a positive change in their symptoms. So, to be on the safe side, there is no harm in increasing your consumption of these nutrients.

Here is a list of food items in which you can find the specific nutrients –

- **Magnesium** – Almonds, pumpkin seeds, peanuts, and spinach
- **Zinc** – Nuts, beans, meat, and shellfish

to another. Now, for the body to produce neurotransmitters, protein is required. Apart from this, the symptoms of impulsivity and hyperactivity are often linked with a rise in the level of sugar in the blood. It can be prevented by increasing protein intake. In fact, this is also why it is advised that your breakfast should be rich in protein. But that's not all. Try different ways in which you can insert some protein in your diet throughout the day. You can have berry smoothies or protein bars, which are not only tasty but also great options for protein intake throughout the day.

Complex carbs, on the other hand, help in reducing the chances of a spike in blood sugar. When you consume more complex carbs, your satiety levels are increased, and you stay full for longer hours. It means your urge to grab on those sugar stuff whenever you feel hungry will reduce. Moreover, consuming complex carbs before going to bed has shown proven effects on better sleep.

So, here are the food items that you should include in your diet to enhance protein intake –

- Lentils and beans
- Poultry and meat products
- Shellfish
- Fish
- Nuts
- Eggs

- **Snack** – Chia seed pudding or fat-free yogurt with berries or fruits of your choice
- **Lunch** – Quinoa with baked chicken or salmon along with a salad of bell peppers, cucumbers, mixed leaves, and toppings can be of your choice but make sure you sprinkle some sunflower seeds on top
- **Snack** – Peanut butter and apple or apple and cinnamon
- **Dinner** – Brown rice with a curry (vegetable or chicken)
- **Dessert** – If you want dessert, then you can have an ounce of dark chocolate, or you can have a warm cuppa of herbal tea before sleeping.

Best Foods for the ADHD Diet

I had given you a rough list of foods that you can eat on this diet, but here, we are going to see the different food items categorized into different nutritional groups. We are also going to see how these particular group of foods help in managing the ADHD symptoms.

Protein & Complex Carbs

ADHD symptoms are relieved to a great extent when you include more protein in your diet. As you might already know, the brain releases certain chemicals in your body, which are known as neurotransmitters, and these chemicals are the ones that are responsible for carrying the messages from one part of the brain medications on your body. They also help in increasing your level of concentration.

- *Complex carbohydrates* – These are one of the healthiest things and should definitely be included in your diet. For this, you have to include fruits and vegetables like kiwi, apples, tangerines, tomatoes, and so on. The complex carbohydrates should be preferably consumed in the latter part of the day, or in dinner because they boost your sleep.
- *Omega-3-fatty acids* – These are another group fo very healthy nutrients that no one should miss. You will find them in fishes like salmon, tuna, and whitefish. They are also present in canola oil, olive oil, brazil nuts, and walnuts. If you think that your diet is not being able to provide you with a sufficient amount of omega-3-fatty acid, then you should consider taking a supplement. As a part of the ADHD management plan, Vayarin is an omega compound that is widely used, and the FDA has also approved it.

Sample Meal Plan

If you are not sure as to where you can start, then here is a sample meal plan that will save your time and also give you a boost of energy for the day –

- **Breakfast** – Whole-wheat toast with some eggs and avocado; some coffee or tea, preferably herbal tea of nutrients, including vitamins and minerals. When you take these supplements, any deficiency that might have formed in your body will be overcome. This plan is supported by those who strongly believe that a shortage of certain nutrients in the body can trigger the symptoms of ADHD.

- **Overall Nutrition** – This plan is based on the assumption of both of the plans mentioned above. You will be eating some foods that are responsible for making you feel good and relieve you from your symptoms, and you will also be eliminating certain food items that are harmful to your symptoms.

Even though the data is relatively limited with respect to the ADHD diet, there are certain things that experts believe after extensive research. They think that following these tips might help the patients get relief from the symptoms. The main thought behind this is that whatever food item boosts brain health is also good for combating ADHD. So, you should eat –

- *A diet rich in protein* – There are so many good sources of protein that you should consume. It includes cheese, beans, nuts, and even meat. Protein should be included in your breakfast to give you a healthy and energy-boosting start, and it should also be included in your snacks. There is a possibility that protein-rich foods help in extending the effect of the ADHD

- Carrots
- Cantaloupe
- Mangoes
- Kiwi
- Kale
- Squash
- Potatoes
- Pineapple
- Peas
- Zucchini
- Watermelon
- Spinach
- Bananas
- Cabbage
- Brussels sprouts
- Lentils
- Lemons
- Sweet corn

Once you practice these eating habits, you will notice a marked difference in your symptoms of inattentiveness and restlessness. Some of the choices that you have under this diet are as follows –

- **Elimination Diets** – When you follow this type of diet, you are consciously choosing not to eat those foods which have been proven to trigger the ADHD symptoms. A list of such food items has already been mentioned above.
- **Supplementation Diets** – In this plan, the goal is to supplement your foods with a variety

- Cherries
- Berries
- Prunes
- Plums
- Pickles and cucumbers
- Oranges
- Tomatoes
- Tea
- Currants
- Peppers
- Peaches
- Nectarines
- Tangerines

Here are some of the foods that you should eat on this diet –

- Beets
- Beans
- Celery
- Dates
- Bean Sprouts
- Lettuce
- Cauliflower
- Onion
- Mushrooms
- Pears
- Honeydew
- Sweet potato
- Grapefruit

In Chapter 3, we studied the causes of ADHD in detail, and there, we saw that additives and colorings in food could increase the chances of developing ADHD. So, the ADHD diet encourages you to eliminate certain things from your diet like –

- Artificial flavorings. One of the most common examples is that of synthetic vanilla.
- Artificial colorings
- Preservatives. Some common examples are TBHQ or tert-Butylhydroquinone, BHT or butylated hydroxytoluene, and BHA or butylated hydroxyanisole.
- Salicylates or any other chemicals that are present in food naturally. Some food items include tomatoes, berries, and apricots.
- Artificial sweeteners. Some common names in this category are sucralose, saccharin, and aspartame.

Now, let us see some of the food items that have been strictly removed from this diet –

- Coffee
- Grapes
- Apricots
- Apples
- Almonds
- Mint flavoring
- Cloves

Chapter 8: What Should You Know About the ADHD Diet?

Most people wonder whether they can improve their power to focus and treat the symptoms of ADHD by eating the right kind of food. Well, to some extent, yes, and that is what we are going to discuss in this chapter. Although there have been no conclusive studies in this field that say that nutritional deficiencies can lead to ADHD, the symptoms can definitely be managed by following a particular diet. There are certain food items that help and certain food items that you shouldn't eat.

What Is ADHD Diet?

Before going into too many details, let us see what the ADHD diet is all about. As you know, ADHD patients tend to become very energetic and hyperactive. This diet helps in alleviating those symptoms. Dr. Benjamin Feingold had suggested some changes to be made in the diet of his patients in the 1970s. These changes showed effectiveness in reducing symptoms of certain conditions like hives, asthma, and behavioral disorders. There have been several variations of the diet that Dr. Feingold created, and research has been done on all of them. There is no conclusive evidence on the reduction of ADHD symptoms. But there have been several patients who claimed that this diet really helped them manage their symptoms and lead a better life.

cytoplasm is the lawn, and the mitochondrion is the power plant. You can also make up a vivid story about a character in the city for added memory power. You can make the character interact with the other elements you have created. Creating a story will help cement the facts in your mind. Make sure to make the story a bit strange in some way so that it can grab the attention of your brain.

- **Mind mapping** – Creating mind maps that link different ideas helps you capitalize on the brain's ability to latch on to geometric shapes. A mind map makes it easier for many people to remember information. Making mind maps are very easy. Simply write your topic anywhere on a piece of paper and then brainstorm important ideas that you get and jot them down anywhere on the paper. Just link them to the ideas that they are connected to when they come to your mind.

Take some time each day to practice these strategies and then try to put them in your everyday life. You can experience an improvement in the effectiveness and efficiency of memorization by using these strategies.

framework to help you remember information. If you are a visual person, you might want to make vivid visuals in your mind. If you are a kinesthetic person, you can incorporate some movements into your mental image. If you think that you are affected by your tactile senses, you can put your sense of touch in your mental image. And, f you think you have a good olfactory sense, then you can incorporate different scents into your mental imagery. These memory techniques work better when they are used together. You can build stronger associations in your mind by incorporating more of these sensory factors into your mental imagery. It can also increase the number of triggers you are leaving behind that can later help you in recalling the information. A multisensory approach can also help you in forming new memories. Try doing it every time you are studying. You can sing it, draw it, read it, write it, or say it. You can do whatever it takes to make it stick.

- **Analogies** – Creating new exciting connections to make the dry facts more personally relevant and meaningful to you is a great way to make things more interesting. For example, when you are trying to memorize the different cell organelles present in the body, consider a cell to be a city and link the function and name of each organelle to the characteristics of the city. For instance, the endoplasmic reticulum is the highway, the

- Folding a piece of paper
- Doodling

Try pulling, pushing, or stretching movements like:
- Pushing against the wall
- Stretching a big elastic band
- Tug of war

Balancing activates the same regions of the brain that also manage attention. Try spinning and balancing movements like:
- Standing on a balance board having rockers under it
- Walking around the room while studying or reading
- Turning around a couple of times in a particular direction and then altering the direction

Try joint compression movements like:
- Bouncing up and down in your chair
- Jumping jacks
- Jumping up and down

- **Capitalize on your natural processing skills** – Everyone has a natural style of processing information. Your superweapons are your natural approaches and your unique set of strengths. You can improve your memory by recognizing and making use of these skills and strengths. When you use your natural processing style, it helps stimulate your senses by making associations in your mind. If you are an auditory person, you can use rhymes, jingles, and songs, which will act as a are not facing the same direction and are mirror images of each other.

- Cross crawl sit-ups: Lie on you back and keep your hands under your head for support. Then, sit up and touch your left elbow to your right knee. Alternate the movement by touching your right elbow to your left knee.
- Karate cross crawl: Use alternate hand and foot to kick while chopping or punching. For instance, when your left foot kicks, your right-hand chops.
- Lazy 8: Trace a large infinity sign in front of your body using one hand. Follow your hand with your eyes. Do it a couple of times and alternate hands.
- Try touching your elbow or hand to your opposite knee.

- **Movements help turn the brain on –** Finding fun and creative ways to include movement in your study time is one of the best ways by which you can stay focused and alert. Try doing any of the following movements given below for at least five minutes before starting your study or work sessions. Also, make sure to incorporate movement breaks into your sessions every fifteen to thirty minutes.

  Try following low concentration, repetitive tasks like the ones given below.
  - Squeezing a ball
  - Rocking

license plates and recite the numbers and letters on them and then taking turns to speak them backward as well.

- **Have your children teach you** – When you can explain how to perform or do something to others, it involves understanding the information and filling it mentally. For instance, if your kid is learning how to dribble a basketball, ask them to teach you how to do it. Teachers also do something similar to this when they pair up students in a class. Doing this allows them to begin working with the facts instantly instead of waiting to be called on.

Top Strategies for Improving Overall Memory

Everyone wants to have a better memory. Here are some simple strategies that you can use to improve your overall memory:

- **Cross lateral movements** – These kinds of movements involve using your legs and hands on opposite sides of your body. You can perform some of these cross-lateral movements for at least 5 minutes every day. This can help you improve your mental alertness and concentration power.
    - o Double doodle: Try drawing a pattern or design using both your hands at the same time. Make sure that the designs

so that they can look at them. Let your child hear them when you say them out loud. Walk with your kid through your house while telling them about the family chores that they need to finish. When you use multisensory strategies, it helps your kids store the information in their minds for a long enough to use it.

- **Encourage active reading** – Highlighting or underlining text and jotting down notes can help children keep the facts in their minds for long enough so that they can answer questions about them. This is why sticky notes and highlighters are so famous nowadays. Asking questions about the text they are reading and reading it out loud can also help with their working memory. Long-term memories can also be formed with the help of these active reading strategies.
- **Play cards** – Easy card games like War, Go Fish, Uno, and Crazy Eights can help strengthen your kid's working memory in 2 ways. Not only do they have to remember and maintain the rules of the game they are playing, but they also need to keep in mind the cards they have and the ones the other players have played.
- **Play games that use visual memory** – Kids can improve their visual memory by playing matching games. You can also try giving your child a page from a magazine and tell them to mark all the instances of the letter "a" or the word "the." It can also be fun to use

one time, like shopping. Forget about the remaining tasks until you have finished shopping.

- **Practice your skills of working memory** – You can create your own brain training programs or use the ones mentioned above. Note down six words that are unrelated to each other. Begin by trying to remember the 1st two words without seeing the paper. Then, as you succeed, add another word to the sequence.

Working memory is used by children all the time to learn things. They need it for things like solving math problems in their heads or following multi-step directions. You can help your kid strengthen their working memory by incorporating some simple strategies in their daily lives. Here are some tips by which you can boost your child's working memory:

- **Help make connections** – Help your kid create links that associate various details and make them memorable. Using fun mnemonics is another great way to grab your kid's attention. Finding ways to link different information also helps in creating and recover long-term memories. It can also help with working memory with which they can hold and compare recent and old memories.
- **Make it multisensory** – Processing information using multiple senses can help improve long-term memory as well as working memory. Note down certain tasks for your kid

visualizing them. Visualize yourself stopping at the grocery store when you are coming home from work and picking up yogurt, bread, cheese, and milk. Try to imagine what it would look like to go to each section of the store. You are more likely to remember all the items you need to purchase at the grocery store if you follow your visualization. It is because images and visuals can be more powerful than words.

- **Develop routines** – When you return from work, start by creating a routine. As soon as you walk through your door, choose a specific place to keep your keys and cell phone. Keep them in the same place every time when you return from work.

- **Use checklists for tasks that have several steps** – Try making a checklist for your first hour at work. It could include several tasks like reviewing yesterday's progress, checking and replying to emails, returning calls, listening to messages, checking with the supervisor for the necessary tasks that need to be finished immediately, etc.

- **Divide large chunks of information into smaller pieces** – Before moving forward to the next instruction, concentrate on one or two of them first. For instance, if you want to get ready to host a party in your house but are stressed and overwhelmed about everything that you need to get done like setting up for the party, cleaning the house, cooking, and shopping. Try concentrating on a single area at

Here are some tips on how you can improve your working memory:

- **Include exercise in your daily routine** – According to a few studies, exercising regularly can improve your working memory. Researchers believe that physical activity and exercise can improve the health of brain cells. It can also reduce stress, help you sleep better, and improve your mood – all of which can indirectly influence your memory and affect your cognitive abilities.
- **Using mindfulness to strengthen your working memory and reduce distractions** – A research conducted by MIT, Massachusetts General Hospital, and Harvard Medical School found that exercising mindfulness techniques daily can improve recall and also allowed the participants to regulate their sensory output and tune out any distractions.
- **Decrease multitasking** – A research conducted at the University of Sussex found that multitasking can decrease particular regions of your brain and is also associated with a reduced attention span. Try finishing the task at hand before moving on to the next task.
- **Try different methods of remembering information** – Making up a rhyme or creating a song might make it easier for you to remember a list of things. Some might also find it easier to remember multiple things by

- You wish to pitch in a conversation. However, you forget what you wanted to say by the time the other person has done speaking.

You require the help of your working memory no matter what you want to do.

You can use a number of services and products (for example, Play Attention and CogMed) to strengthen your working memory and train your brain. Several studies have revealed that such products and services can improve your working memory; however, the benefits might not last beyond the training session. Other studies have, however, shown that if you commit to training your brain, it can significantly improve your working memory.

The first step to strengthening your working memory is by understanding your own limitations and knowing how memory works. It does not mean you can excuse yourself by just saying that you are sorry. It means you can compensate for forgetting by developing and using certain strategies. People who have ADHD often try to keep things in order by using reminder systems. They might keep a list of things they need to buy at the grocery store or keep a running to-do list on a notepad app on their tablet or phone. They might also use a calendar app or a timer to remind them of their appointments.

Tips to Boost Working Memory

write, or read. It helps us to stay engaged and focused on a task. Working memory is also important for students. Recent research conducted in the United Kingdom with around 3000 junior high and grade-school students revealed that struggles in school were caused mostly due to weak working memory and not because of low IQ. Studies also showed that almost all the students who had a poor working memory scored less in math and reading comprehension.

Here are some examples of how your daily life is affected by weak working memory:

- Your inability to follow through on projects and your disorganization causes you to miss deadlines at work.
- In order to retain information, you have to reread something multiple times.
- You plan to work from the comfort of your house; however, you don't remember to bring the items that you require with you.
- You get distracted and forget about the first project, and so have several unfinished projects.
- While having a conversation with someone, you forget what the other person has just said and so have difficulty following a conversation.
- Even when you were just told the directions to a place, you tend to get lost easily.
- You keep losing your wallet, cell phone, or keys.

number that another person can store in his working memory. Studies have revealed that young children can hold only one or two things in their working memory as they have limited working memory skills. It continues to develop until one reaches the age of fifteen. However, not everyone has the same capacity for working memory, and it doesn't develop at the same pace for everyone. Some people can accommodate more items in their mental shelf than others.

Scientists don't agree on the number of information "bytes" that the brain can hold. According to some, it's just around four, while others claim that it's as many as seven items. Several studies have also been conducted, which showed that one's working memory could be strengthened and improved. You can increase your capacity of working memory by grouping things together. For instance, a phone number generally consists of ten digits; however, we often divide the number into three separate groups. It helps us to remember the ten-digit number by making use of only three working memory slots. Working memory is similar to plastic – trainable, movable, and flexible. It is just like our muscles and can be improved with the help of training and exercise.

When Do We Use Working Memory?

Working memory is used by us in various situations every day. We use it to follow multi-step directions, do mental math, follow a conversation, organize, plan, impulsive behaviors, and improve their ability to focus.

What Is Working Memory?

The term "working memory" and "short-term memory" are often used interchangeably. You might have heard either of these terms before. The terms refer to a "temporary storage system" that is located in the brain to store various thoughts and facts while you are performing a task or solving a problem. It, thus, allows you to store information and thoughts temporarily in your mind so that you can use them whenever you need them to finish a task. Working memory helps you to hold facts and thoughts for long enough so that you can use it in a short while, remember what to do next, and concentrate on your task at hand.

You can consider working memory to be a shelf in your brain. For example, you have to go to the supermarket because you need bread, eggs, and milk. While you are shopping for these things in the supermarket, you suddenly remember that you have to buy cereal as well. So you go to the cereal aisle. However, having to buy eggs falls off your mental shelf as you focus on buying the cereal. You come back home with bread, milk, and cereal and realize that you have forgotten to buy the eggs.

The total number of things that you can accommodate on your mental shelf might be different than the

Chapter 7: How to Sharpen Your Memory When You Have ADHD?

People with ADHD often suffer from executive function (EF) deficits with some of the most profound impairments linked with working memory, fluid intelligence, processing speed, planning, vigilance, and response inhibition. These EF deficits can be seen as a sign of lower intelligence and can lead to reduced self-esteem, decreased professional or academic achievements, and reduced income. It is thought that the intelligence deficits seen in people who have ADHD are caused because of impairments in higher-order cognitive processes (like working memory) and not due to direct impairment of cognitive abilities.

A majority of people who have ADHD or ADD have problems with working memory. Occasionally most of us forget important dates or lose our keys or leave our wallet in the refrigerator. You might think that these happen because you are inattentiveness. However, when these turn into habits, you might have a poor working memory associated with ADHD. They might have problems with differentiating between important and unimportant cues, organizing, focusing, and recalling things. It might be hard for them to get started on tasks, and might become forgetful and get distracted easily. It is often impossible and frustrating for them to follow lengthy multiple-step directions. Sharpening your working memory can help strengthen a person's problem-solving skills, control

You can even set the timer to go off after every hour to let you know that an hour has passed.

- You need to bring more structure into your life. Make it a habit to plan your day before going to bed. So, create a list of things that need to be done the next day and then prioritize them. You can also assign a particular time span to each of these tasks to make it more organized.

- Learn to say no and create healthy boundaries. Don't bite more than you can eat. Stress is often raised when you overbook yourself.

- No matter how busy your life is, learn to take breaks from time to time. Make it a resolution to go out with your friends every weekend at a dinner or a movie night. You can even plan your weekends around your hobbies or go for a drive towards the countryside.

By now, you must have learned that ADHD can make people stressed out and worry about petty things. It is not easy to lead a life with ADHD weighing down upon your shoulders. But if you follow these tips, your life will gradually become more manageable.

But there are ways in which you can reduce this stress and get a grip on your life –

- Stress is created when you keep blaming and guilt-tripping yourself every time you forget something or miss a deadline. Stop doing this right now. Remind yourself that you have ADHD, and it is in your neurobiology to forget things. If you are not seeking treatment for ADHD, then visit a specialist right away. You can even join an internet forum or local support group to talk and listen to other people who have ADHD. This will help you acknowledge the fact that you have ADHD. The more you do these things, the more you will see that you are not the only one in this world to be dealing with these problems. This realization, in turn, will reduce your stress.
- Practice physical activity. It can be anything – it can be a ten-minute brisk walk around the block or some free-hand exercises at home. When you do some physical activity, the brain releases a particular chemical known as serotonin. Serotonin functions opposite to cortisol (the hormone responsible for stress). Moreover, your body's threshold of withstanding stress also increases the more you exercise.
- The concept of time is seen as a fluid thing by most ADHD patients. Practice wearing a watch at all times or keep a table clock on your desk.

- Refrain from consuming any type of caffeine at least four hours before going to bed.
- Don't take a nap about four hours before you go to bed.
- Maintain a fixed time for going to bed every day.
- Start a bedtime routine that helps you to relax. The routine should not be too elaborate.
- If you cannot change your stimulant medication, then you should at least try to take these medications in the earlier part of the day.
- Make sure your bedroom is appropriately dark and quiet for you to have a good sleeping atmosphere.
- Don't spend too much time looking at screens before bedtime.

Stress

The symptoms of ADHD can easily trigger you to become stressed – it is quite common, and it happens with everyone. The list of things that can cause you to become stressed is endless. A constant state of stress is what many ADHD patients complain about. Slowing down in life is a big battle, and they cannot focus on important things. Additional stress is created when they constantly miss their deadlines or feel guilty about missing those deadlines. It also leads to an increased amount of frustration that keeps accumulating.

- ADHD medication often consists of stimulants, and one of the side-effects of these medications is that they hamper the sleeping pattern. They tend t make you feel more energetic, and so you feel like you are awake at all times. Conditions become worse when you have chocolate, coffee, tea, or any other source of caffeine.
- Keeping a schedule is difficult for ADHD patients. They have a hard time dealing with distractions in their day to day life. Even when they go to bed, they have all these thoughts running in their head that makes it difficult for them to calm their brain. Since they cannot reach this relaxed state of mind, they find it difficult to fall asleep.
- ADHD patients also have other disorders at times like mood disorders, anxiety, and depression, and all of them add to the problem of not getting proper sleep.

The first thing that you should do is inform your doctor because sometimes, all you need is a change in your medications or your dosage, and you will be able to sleep well. Also, your sleeplessness might not be as simple as it means. It can be due to some other underlying reason, and only a doctor will be able to tell you that for sure. But if all other causes have been examined and ruled out, then you have to inculcate some healthy habits and manage your ADHD-related sleeping problem –

Once someone has developed substance abuse problems, the treatment process is extensive and difficult, so every effort has to be made to prevent the problem altogether. For this, you should start talking to the kids from a young age about avoiding illicit drugs and the dangers of substance abuse. For adults, if you want to set yourself free from the habit of self-medication, then you should exercise daily because it really helps. When you exercise, it helps in stimulating the ADHD and prevents you from getting bored. Your brain becomes more vulnerable when you are bored, so it is important to keep yourself engaged.

Sleep Problem

ADHD has been found to cause sleep problems in patients of every age. There was a study in 2006 that found out that children who have ADHD often show symptoms of daytime sleepiness, whereas children without ADHD don't (Samuele Cortese, 2006). There was another study that showed that sleeping disordered breathing was found in 50% of the kids diagnosed with ADHD (Natali Golan, 2004). There have also been studies that show periodic leg movement and restless leg syndrome, both of which disrupt sleep, are more prevalent in kids who have ADHD than those who don't (Avi Sadeh, 2006).

But the most common question that people have is that why does ADHD cause sleep problems? Well, there are a number of reasons behind this, and they are as follows –

you feel think is right for you. The whole idea of journaling is to be comfortable with your own thoughts and writing them down. You don't necessarily have to do it in a fancy way. But if you do like to take things up a notch and be artistic, then it is completely your choice. You can even note down all your thoughts that you want to discuss with your therapist on your next session.

- Lastly, have patience because treating anxiety is not an overnight thing. It takes consistent effort and weeks for you to figure out which line of treatment is working for you.

Substance Abuse

There are several instances where patients of ADHD have been found to have substance abuse problems. In fact, among the patients who are admitted to a treatment center for drug and alcohol abuse, 25% have ADHD. But why does substance abuse and ADHD go hand in hand? Well, for starters, most patients turn to substance abuse to get a hold on their life. ADHD brains have reduced amounts of dopamine, and using drugs or alcohol increases that level. Moreover, alcoholism and ADHD both are conditions that have the tendency to run in families. So, if an ADHD child has a parent who also had ADHD and alcohol abuse problems, then the child is very much susceptible to developing the same as well.

you some medication that will help you sleep. You can also try meditation because that often helps in these situations. Another thing to try is to maintain a fixed time of waking up in the morning and going to sleep at night. But never make the mistake of taking meds without consulting your doctor.

- Follow a fixed schedule. Completing tasks on your to-do list is one of the biggest hurdles of ADHD patients, and when tasks remain incomplete, it causes anxiety. But this can be prevented if you make a schedule and abide by it. When you prepare this schedule, don't make it too tight. If the schedule becomes too hard to follow, then you will always be rushing to complete things and get anxious in the process. So, set goals that are realistic.

- Here too, I would like to remind you that exercising regularly can actually help you in reducing your anxiety. It has been proven in different studies (Elizabeth Anderson, 2013). Even if you have a busy schedule, make sure you do at least half an hour of some form of physical activity. If you haven't had an exercise routine in your life, then I would advise you to start small. Work your way up slowly, and then you can practice a couple of intense workouts if you feel like it.

- Journaling is a very effective way to relieve anxiety. It helps you take the stress off your mind. There are no rules when it comes to journaling – you can do it in whichever way

Having anxiety attacks is much more than that. It can make you feel frightened to unnatural levels; you will feel distressed and uneasy even when you are under normal circumstances. It has been found that among the adults who have ADHD, about 40-60% also have anxiety (Hechtman, 2008).

There are different patterns in which anxiety can show itself in ADHD patients – it can be in the form of behavioral changes, cognitive changes, mood swings, or any physical activity. When anxiety strikes, the symptoms are quite paralyzing, and resuming normal lie can become a real struggle. Whenever a person with ADHD thinks that there might be a negative outcome to a situation, they start avoiding things. Anxiety also hampers with proper decision-making skills and leads to procrastination. So, how can an ADHD patient deal with anxiety? Here's how –

- The first step is to find what your triggers are. Some people can pinpoint events that cause them to become anxious – it can be as simple as receiving phone calls to complex things like public speaking. Your path to managing your anxiety will become much easier once you identify the events that are triggering you.
- The next thing to ensure is that you are getting enough sleep. Anxiety is often triggered when the ADHD brain does not get proper rest. Make it a resolution to sleep for 7-8 hours at night. In case you cannot sleep after going to bed, you should consult your doctor. He/She might give

during eating. But when you eat, if you focus on truly enjoying the food rather than anticipating the next move and gulping down more and more, it helps. After every five minutes, check with yourself whether you like the food or not. Don't think about the next course of the meal but focus on what you are eating now.

- Lastly, even if you make a mistake and end up overeating once, don't beat yourself too much. If self-loathing and yelling at your own self would have solved everything, then you would have overcome compulsive eating long back. So, if you slip, just forget the past, learn from your mistakes, and start your healthy eating plan again.

Anxiety

Before we move on to how anxiety is caused because of ADHD, you need to understand that ADHD and anxiety are not the same. They are two different disorders. But how will you understand that you have anxiety apart from having symptoms of ADHD? Well, it's quite simple really – if you are into constant worrying that is ruining your day-to-day life and also preventing you from doing normal things, then you are suffering from anxiety. Some people even complain that having anxiety has made them feel that they are always on edge.

Remember that all of us feel anxious from time to time, but that doesn't classify it as an anxiety disorder.

moves that come naturally. It will give you an energy boost and also uplift your mood. Even if you are not feeling like it, make yourself get up and walk for ten minutes or so. By the end of those ten minutes, you will feel the tension leaving your body, you will have greater energy levels, and your subjective hunger will reduce too.

- The next thing that we are going to discuss is quite useful – schedule your eating times. When you have ADHD, your brain is often not aware of what you feel. The brain always tries to stay ahead of others, and this same tendency is what makes you feel disconnected from everything else. When you are too focused on something else, you don't have a sense of time, and you forget to eat. It, in turn, makes you more hungry, and you overeat. But setting reminders for eating can solve this problem. Make it a resolution to eat something after every three to four hours, even if it is a snack. This will stimulate your brain and will also relieve you from the restlessness.

- Even after you follow all these tips, you still have to teach yourself how you can stop eating. For this, fix a particular serving size and follow it. When you are eating, concentrate on how you feel and analyze each state of feeling that you are experiencing. This is called mindful eating, and this is going to help you a lot with respect to binge eating. Binge eating is mostly the result of the pleasure that we anticipate exercise schedule or making healthier meals daily.

- Now, let us talk about food temptations. ADHD patients are not good at showing resistance, and so you should avoid doing it altogether. Everyone has a particular type of food that they tend to overeat. Find out what is yours and then keep that specific food item out of your reach. Don't buy things that you know you might end up overeating. I am not telling you to altogether opt-out of eating ice-cream, but I am asking you to do so infrequently. If you keep ice-cream in the fridge, battling that temptation to grab the ice-cream tub, the first chance you get would be hard. So, if you really want to have ice-cream at some point, you can just go out and have some.

- Like I said before, people with ADHD often interpret boredom as hunger and overeat. So, you have to stimulate your brain and keep it engaged so that you don't feel bored. For this, you have to set a limit for a daily stimulation dose and make sure you meet the minimum limit every day. The more exciting tasks you do, the less you will be searching for amusement in food. I would like to remind you that watching television doesn't fall into this category of exciting tasks. Instead, TV can make you want to overeat, and it does not provide much brain stimulation as well.

- Don't forget to exercise. You don't have to perform any heavy exercise, but just a few dopamine in the brain is also lowered when they have ADHD. Dopamine is responsible for giving your body the 'feel-good' feeling, and binge eating raises the level dopamine. So, automatically, it is quite natural for you to want to binge eat.

As you know, impulsivity is one of the main symptoms of ADHD, and this impulsivity applies to all spheres of the person's life, including eating. In fact, it has been found that compulsive eating or binge eating as a habit is five times more common in those who have ADHD. The cognitive functions of people with ADHD are very poor, and they cannot interpret the meaning of things like all of us. So, they cannot understand what other people are trying to tell them, and similarly, they cannot understand what their bodies are trying to say to them. Thus, when they feel bored or upset, they think that the feeling is because they are hungry. So, to combat that feeling, they reach out to food.

So, if you are facing the same issue in your life, then here are some ways in which you can combat it –

- An ADHD brain can be put to good use too, for example, to lose weight. When people have ADHD, it is not that their brain is not sharp; it just doesn't know when to stop. So, in order to lose weight, your focus should not be on eating less but on something more fruitful. You can place your focus on getting engaged in a new

Chapter 6: Living With ADHD

Almost every aspect of life is affected by ADHD. But there are some tips that you can follow in order to make living with the symptoms much more manageable. Everything around you might seem chaotic, but once you follow these tips, things will start falling into place.

ADHD in adults can make their lives seem overwhelming at all times. Whether it is the work deadlines that you have to complete or family gatherings that you cannot afford to miss, everything starts to seem like a burden. And dealing with this feeling day in and day out is hectic and stressful. There will be hurdles in every area of your life. It is going to lay a massive impact on your relationships, both personal and professional.

The quality of life is reduced to a great extent. But if you want to know about the specific aspects of your life that are affected by ADHD and how you can minimize the problems, keep reading.

Binge Eating

Binge eating or compulsive eating is one of the direct results of ADHD. It is mainly because the patients of ADHD struggle very much whenever they have to set some kind of discipline or limitation on their habits. And, eating is one such habit that tends to go out of control in ADHD. Moreover, in adults, the level of

So, these were the most common types of treatment options that are there for ADHD. But here is something that you should know – about 75% of the ADHD patients suffer from at least one other psychiatric problem during their lifetime. It can be substance use disorders, bipolar disorder, depressive disorder, anxiety disorder, or antisocial personality disorder. If the co-existing condition of the patient is severe, then the treatment for that is started first, and then ADHD is administered.

Remember that the goal of your treatment is not only to help you manage the symptoms but also to help you improve your overall quality of life.

problems dealing with social settings. So, situations are created during the sessions where the child has to do role-play and learn how they should react in that situation. The process is really fun, and the children get to learn a lot of important things.

CBT

CBT stands for Cognitive Behavioral Therapy, and this therapy can be very fruitful in adults as well. The therapist will walk you through the process, and you will learn to change your perspective of things. It, in turn, will help you improve your behavior in different situations. The therapist uses several strategies to change your thoughts about various incidents and how you react to them. CBT can be done in a group or individually.

Nowadays, CBT programs have become developed because they teach adults a lot of things – managing time, overcoming hurdles in executive functions, and also stress management. The behavioral skills that are imparted by CBT have been found to be more useful for the patients. In fact, research has pointed out that irrespective of whether the patient is under medication or not, CBT alone can do wonders for minimizing ADHD symptoms. Interpersonal self-regulation is another benefit of CBT, along with several aspects of self-management. All the irrational beliefs that the patient might have are challenged through CBT, and then with the help of proper discussions, those beliefs are negated.

Psychoeducation

This type of therapy can be helpful for people of all ages. The ultimate motive of psychoeducation is to simplify the idea of ADHD understandable to the patient. The patients are made aware of the different symptoms that they might face and also the effects of those symptoms on their day-to-day activities. This kind of therapy helps the patient to adjust to ADHD and cope with it while living a normal and well-balanced life.

Behavior Therapy

This therapy is mainly designed for children with ADHD. The therapy usually involves both parents and teachers as well. The children are introduced to the concept of rewards. Then that is used to monitor and control their behavior. So, parents are asked what kind of behavior do they want to teach their child? For example, some children might not be cleaning their room, so the goal of the therapy would be to teach the child to keep their room tidy. So, if the child follows through and does what he/she is asked to, then they will be given a reward in the end for their good behavior. It is how good behavior is encouraged in the child. When teachers are involved in this therapy, it is mainly about teaching the child different types of structural activities. No matter how little the progress is, you should always encourage your child and be positive so that their motivation stays intact.

There is another part of behavior therapy, which is called social skills training. ADHD kids often face

these medications include dizziness, headaches, low blood pressure, and drowsiness. But if you are taking these medications, make sure you don't miss the dose, and even if you do, you need to call your doctor immediately.

Lastly, we are going to see how anti-depressants work for ADHD patients. People who have both depression and ADHD are usually the ones taking these. They help keep the aggressiveness in check and also control hyperactivity. They have quite significant effects on improving attention. When these drugs are prescribed to children, it is noticed that they automatically become disciplined and take directions easily. But you have to keep in mind that when compared to stimulants, they don't work that well. The primary mechanism of the working of these drugs is that they increase the levels of certain neurochemicals in the brain. Some of these chemicals are dopamine, serotonin, and norepinephrine. But if someone has epilepsy or a history of seizures, then they can't take Bupropion. Also, anyone having a history of bipolar disorder is refrained from using anti-depressants.

Can Therapy Help?

ADHD can be treated with the help of therapy in children, adults, and teenagers. Moreover, if someone is facing problems like anxiety or panic attacks, then that can be addressed with therapy too. In this section, you will learn about the major types of therapies that are mostly used to treat ADHD.

anti-depressants, antipsychotics, and blood pressure meds.
- You have an intense history of alcohol and drug abuse and dependency.
- You have shown symptoms of allergic reactions to any medicine in the past.
- You suffer from some medical problems related to blood pressure, kidney, jaundice, liver problems, mental health problems, seizures, glaucoma, and heart problems.
- You are planning to become pregnant, or you are nursing, or you are currently pregnant.
- You take any over-the-counter medication, herbal medication, or dietary supplements.
- You frequently have suicidal thoughts or get irritated too easily.

After discussing all the factors, if your doctor advises you that non-stimulants can indeed work for you, then you need to make sure that you take your medication daily as recommended by him/her. To find out whether the drug is working for you or not, your doctor might also prescribe some tests for you. Now, let us see how or why blood pressure drugs can be helpful in case of treating ADHD. It is mainly because these medicines have been found to help with the symptoms of ADHD and also have fewer side effects. It has not yet been found as to how do the medications for high blood pressure help ADHD patients, but it is probably because of the soothing and calming effect they bring on some parts of the brain. But some commonly seen side effects of taking

- Have depression and take a particular drug called MAOI or monoamine oxidase inhibitor. Some common examples of this drug include tranylcypromine and phenelzine.
- Have been diagnosed with a specific eye condition known as narrow-angle glaucoma. This condition is quite dangerous because it can lead to complete blindness by putting unnatural pressure on the eyes.
- Suffer from liver or jaundice problems
- Are allergic to this medication or any of its ingredients in particular

Similarly, you shouldn't take the medicine Clonidine if you have faced some sort of allergic reaction after taking it.
On the other hand, Guanfacine shouldn't be taken by those who –

- Already consume other meds having guanfacine in it
- Are allergic to the medication or any of its components in particular.

So, here are some final thoughts on things you should keep in mind before taking non-stimulants. You need to inform your doctor if you have any of these conditions –

- You take any other medication for other health problems that require you to have sedatives, are also used in the treatment of ADHD because the ingredients of these medications are somewhat similar to those of non-stimulants.

So, let us talk about the non-stimulants that are ADHD-specific. One of the most common ones in this category is Atomoxetine, and it can be used for children, teenagers, and adults. This particular medication is mainly responsible for controlling the levels of norepinephrine and giving it a slight boost. The use of this medication helps the patient manage their hyperactive behavior and concentrate better. Two of the other medicines in this category that are approved for use in children are Guanfacine ER and Clonidine ER, and they can be administered to children between the age group of six to seventeen. They can be prescribed to adults as well. The use of these medicines helps improve memory, attention power, and impulse control.

There are certain advantages of using non-stimulants as compared to stimulants. Firstly, the non-stimulants won't lead to problems like loss of appetite, insomnia, or agitation. They are not addictive and won't cause substance abuse problems. Moreover, when compared to stimulants, these medications are much smoother, and their effect lasts for a more extended period. But some people shouldn't be taking non-stimulants. I am going to break it down to you in detail below – *Atomoxetine is a drug that shouldn't be taken by people who –*

people who do not have it. Well, the answer is no. When you follow the dosage prescribed by your doctor, you should be fine and not have any substance abuse problems. In fact, there is no proof that ADHD meds lead to substance abuse. It has been noticed that adults who undergo the treatment of ADHD are the ones who do not encounter any substance abuse problems as compared to the higher percentage of people giving in to substance abuse when they have an untreated ADHD.

Non-Stimulants

If the doctor decides that the patient should not be taking stimulants, then they prescribe non-stimulants. Sometimes, doctors give both stimulants and non-stimulants.

Non-stimulants are of three different types –

- **ADHD-Specific** – As you can understand from the term, these non-stimulants have been specially designed for ADHD, and the FDA has also approved them for ADHD.
- **Anti-depressants** – The next type of non-stimulants are the anti-depressants, which help in stabilizing some neurochemicals and alleviate the symptoms. These medicines are also prescribed to those who deal with both ADHD and one of the following – mood disorders, anxiety, or depression.
- **Blood Pressure Medicines** – Yes, medicines used for regulation of blood pressure

from time to time for follow-ups is very necessary. It will help to keep a check on whether you have any side effects. It will also let you know whether the meds are working properly. After a while, your doctor might also put you off the meds for a while. It is to ensure that your body's reaction to it can be monitored. It will help the doctor understand whether you still need to continue the meds or not. The doctor might also suggest taking off from the meds periodically for short periods so that your body doesn't become fully dependent on them. If you don't do this, then the most common consequence is that you might need a higher dose.

Sometimes the symptoms seem to be going crazier, and that's when changing the time or dosage of meds is rewarding in most cases. Some of the most commonly seen side effects include panic, anxiety, jitteriness, dry mouth, sleeplessness, mood swings, and headache.

But you should also keep in mind that these stimulant medications are not suitable for everyone. In some cases, patients suffer from too many side effects to continue the meds. Also, you might be prescribed something other than stimulants if you have other conditions like psychosis, high blood pressure, anxiety, bipolar disorder, Tourette's syndrome, or problems related to substance abuse.

The most commonly asked question among patients and their families is whether the medications of ADHD can lead to substance abuse problems in because you are not taking the right medicines for yourself. The medicines are different for adults and children, and there are only a few drugs that are meant for both.

So, the different types of drugs that are used in the treatment of adult ADHD are mentioned below.

Stimulants

When it comes to the treatment of ADHD, one of the first things that doctors prescribe are stimulants, and the reason is that these drugs tend to show the best results on patients. In most cases, the initial dosage is low, and then after every week, the dosage is slowly increased. With time, you will reach a point where you try a perfect balance of therapy and meds and limit your overall side-effects and also learn how to keep your symptoms in check.

In the case of adults, the most commonly prescribed medications include Daytrana, Adderall XR, Focalin XR, Concerta, and Vyvanse, and all of these are categorized as long-acting stimulants. The effect of these medications last for at least ten to fourteen hours at a stretch, and so, they are enough to get a person through the day. Another benefit is that the patient does not have to remember taking too many pills or frequent pills. Moreover, with these meds, there is a gradual improvement in symptoms—it helps the patient merge in with their new lifestyle.

Once you have accustomed yourself to the medicine and your dosage has been fixed, going to the doctor

Chapter 5: Treatments for ADHD

Both therapy and medication are used for the treatment of ADHD. Basically, a combination of both these things is what the patient truly needs to make the symptoms manageable. With time, the patient will realize that the symptoms are no longer so difficult to deal with in their day-to-day life.

What Are the Medications Used in ADHD?

In this section, we are going to talk about the major types of medications used in the treatment of ADHD. But I would like to remind you once again that these medications are in no way going to cure ADHD permanently because ADHD cannot be cured. Yes, you can alleviate the symptoms and make your life easier, but the condition will remain with you throughout life. Once you start taking the meds, you can readily divulge into new skills, be attentive, feel calmer, and also feel less impulsive. The dosage of medications also differs depending on the types of medicines that you have been prescribed. Some of them are meant to be taken daily, while others are supposed to be taken only when you have some important work.

Also, which medication is going to work for you is something that you will understand after a bit of trial and error. In the beginning, you might find that the medication is not working properly – that's probably

Once all of these processes are complete, the doctor will look through all the conclusive findings and determine whether the patient has ADHD or not.

- Is the family of the patient capable of giving him/her the care they need at this moment?

Once the initial interviews with the caregiver or the family members are over, the specialists will then talk with the patient. The patient will always have his/her questions about the situation. Listening to their side of the story is equally essential for diagnosis. It can be quite a challenging process, especially if the person is not open to the idea of seeking the help of mental health professionals. The age of the patient is a huge determining factor as far as the perspective is concerned. But this step is vital because it will make the patient more open to the idea of treatment, and they will gradually become comfortable with the process.

Medical History and Physical Exam

Now, no matter what diagnostic assessment we are talking about, it can never be complete without checking what the overall health of the person is. It is even more critical if the person has started showing the symptoms only recently. If the symptoms did not show themselves gradually and were rather sudden, then the cause might not be ADHD in the first place.

The medical history of the patient will be demanded as part of the routine process. So, if the patient has any pre-existing medical conditions like asthma, allergies, epilepsy, and so on, then they have to declare it. The specialist might also ask questions related to the presence of psychiatric illness in the family.

Once this is done, we move on to the last test that is done in this step – the memory test. Although, apart from the memory test, some other small general tests are also done. The memory test examines not only the patient's long-term memory skills but also short-term memory. The tests measure their distractibility, delayed memory, retrieval from memory, and auditory and visual memory.

Clinical Interviews

The second step in the process of diagnosis is the round of clinical interviews. These interviews are constructed to get information about the patient's educational history, family, and other personal facts. Detailed histories are collected not only from the patient but also from the other close people in his/her life. Everyone might have a different perspective, and once this interview round is over, all the perspectives are arranged in order to form a complete picture.

Some of the information that is asked to the caregivers or parents of the patient are as follows –

- How have the symptoms been progressing ever since they showed themselves?
- When or under what circumstances did the symptoms first appear?
- Under what settings are the patients facing functional difficulties, and how severe are they?
- What impact are the symptoms having on the family and the patient?

other disorders. One of the prime requirements of these tests is a consistent level of mental effort, which is something ADHD patients struggle with. The tests require a person to be fast-paced, attentive, and solid memory skills, all of which are not present in ADHD patients. Moreover, in most of these tests, the instructions are not repeated more than once. So, it is because of these tests that the intellectual functioning of a person can be judged.

Next, the achievement tests are usually designed to judge the person's skills in specific subjects. It can be mathematics or even oral language. Sometimes, diagnosing ADHD becomes easier because kids who have ADHD have a specific performance pattern in these tests. That pattern can then be used by experts to make a future diagnosis as well. Scores are usually high when a particular task does not require the person to engage in sustained effort. On the contrary, scores are low when the task requires sustained mental effort and concentration.

As you know that ADHD patients have trouble paying attention, and so, the next test done during the diagnosis are the tests of attention. Even though it might sound like an easy test for you, it is not. There are four different aspects of attention, namely, sustained attention, alternating attention, selective attention, and divided attention. In order to find what the weaknesses and strengths of a patient are, all the aspects of attention are tested.

There will be checklists and questionnaires regarding the behavior of the patient – this is basically a self-report. In case the patient is a child, a 'report by other' is also done, and in that case, the questionnaires and checklists will have to be answered by someone who spends a lot of time with the child. Once all of these reports have been completed, a score is calculated. This score is the point of comparison to find out what is ordinary and what stands out and might be a possible symptom of ADHD. Several standardized rating scales are also used by specialists in order to evaluate the information. One of the most important parts of the comprehensive assessment of a child or adult is the behavioral checklist. But these reports cannot solely diagnose ADHD. They are just a part of the process.

After the behavioral checklists, it is time for the intelligence tests, which are also very crucial. There are some standard tests that are done first, and then once the findings arrive, some special tests might also be done depending on the findings. Tests of daily functioning, achievement tests, and intelligence tests are some of the common tests that are done. These can further include personality tests, memory tests, and symptoms checklists. There are two basic components of intelligence, and these are judged by these tests. These components are – the ability of a person to learn from what happened before and the ability to adapt to new situations. Basically, when these intelligence tests are conducted, the specialists are looking for any inconsistencies in the cognitive and behavioral patterns that are usually present in

problem might lead to a denied diagnosis of those who truly have ADHD. So, when someone is making a decision regarding the diagnosis of ADHD, they should be considering both sides of the story.

Here is something else that should be kept in mind – sometimes, patients are overpathologized by the diagnosis. That is not what an ideal situation should be. The ultimate aim of diagnosis is to give the necessary help to the person. The diagnosis should not convince the person that he/she is a failure, or it should not give them an excuse to give up on their lives. The diagnosis should be the first step towards selecting the most effective form of treatment for that person.

Step-By-Step Guide to Diagnosing ADHD

Here I am going to guide you through a step-by-step approach to ADHD diagnosis –

Social, Academic, and Emotional Functioning Assessment

This is the first step in ADHD diagnosis. The different aspects of life are evaluated, and this holds true for both adults and children. Once a detailed assessment report is made, it will be compared to kids who do not have ADHD to see what is abnormal and what is normal.

aspect of their life. So, do not trust anything that the patient has said unless and until you have cross-referenced it with something else. That is why diagnosis is advised to be done in a combination of feedback tests from colleagues, school records, and families.

The society that we live is provided us with a daily amount of stimulation that can lead to the formation of ADHD like symptoms. So, at any particular point in time, there is a lot of things on your plate competing to get your attention. On top of all that, you might also feel stressed because of your personal relationships. If someone lives in a dysfunctional family or works at a chaotic office, then it can not only cause inattention but also cause mood disorder.

The comorbidity rates in the case of ADHD are so high that it often causes a lot of confusion. It causes distraction, and people are no longer sure whether it is ADHD or not. There might be some obvious disorders in a person that is easily diagnosable, but he/she might also have ADHD that is subtle. In such a case, the diagnosis of ADHD is overlooked. Only a very patient diagnostician with an informed approach can rule it as ADHD if they keep an eye on all the other co-existing problems.

Another challenge that is faced is that certain drugs that are used in the treatment of ADHD have a tendency to induce addiction. So, there are people who tend to fake ADHD just because they want to get hold of those drugs. At the same time, this same some people are not diagnosed in their childhood years. The symptoms are not expressed in the same manner in children and adults. The reason behind the complexity of the diagnosis process of ADHD is that it depends on a lot of historical data of the patient, and all this information needs to be accurate. The process of collecting all that data and ensuring that it is correct can be quite challenging and also a tedious task. AHD can develop anytime after the age of 12. And if the person who is going to the specialist is already an adult, then he is going have a lot of trouble remembering things that happened when he was 12 years old.

A multi-source assessment has to be made to make the results concrete. Thus, different sources have to be used. Some of the examples include – history of employment records from school, any interviews that the person might have attended, and so on. So, going through all the available records and looking for diagnostic clues everywhere is how a proper diagnosis is made. The developmental problems are going to become even more commonplace if the person has a family history of consistent ADHD. Any member of the family having ADHD completely changes the game because then the genetic factor is added.

Moreover, if someone does have ADHD, then they do not have the best memory, and thus, their accounts of what happened earlier cannot simply be trusted. When asked, they might say that they are facing problems in some aspect of their life when, in reality, nothing like that is happening there but in some other

Your next step should be to call up your health insurance company. Sometimes these treatments are not covered, and at other times, they are. You can also ask them for names of specialists if the treatment is covered under the package. Once you have narrowed down to the prospective specialists, call them up, ask them for how long they have been practicing, and any other questions that you might have.

Here are some of the things that you can ask –

- What is their usual line of treatment for ADHD?
- Have they worked with children before, and if yes, then for how long?
- How can you make an appointment with the doctor?

Before you find the person who is a perfect fit for you, it is quite natural that you will have to do a bit of hit and trial. The person that you finally choose should be someone who has a welcoming attitude, and you think that you will be comfortable talking to them. If, after a few appointments, you or your child are still struggling with building a bond, then I think it is time that you look for another therapist.

Diagnostic Challenges

As already discussed, there are a lot of challenges related to ADHD diagnosis. The major one being that

give you therapy and counseling sessions. If you are seeking a diagnosis for your child, then it is better that you visit a psychiatrist who already has experience working with kids in the past.

- **Psychologist** – When a health professional seeks a degree in psychology, they are referred to as a psychologist. They can offer you with different types of therapies like behavioral therapy and social skills therapy. They can even assist you in testing your child's IQ and, after that, take the necessary steps to mitigate the symptoms. In a few places, psychologists also have the power to prescribe medications, but in other places, psychologists are not always allowed to prescribe. In that case, they will ask you to visit a doctor who can prescribe meds.

Now, we come to the question – how are we to find a specialist who meets all our criteria and is right for us? This person should be someone you are comfortable with. Sometimes you might not find the right person at once. You will have to make appointments with some of them, visit them, and then decide for yourself whether you like them or not. That is why it is advised that you go to your primary care doctor, get an initial diagnosis, and also ask him/her for a reference. If you know someone who has ADHD, then you can also ask them for a reference. If it's your child who you think has ADHD, then you can also contact the school and ask them for a reference suitable for a child.

symptoms back to the earlier years and help you think whether you faced them even before or not.

- **How long do you have the symptoms?** – This is somewhat related to the previous question, but here is something that you should know – if anyone is to be diagnosed with ADHD, the symptoms should be persisting for at least six months. It is only after that the specialist can rule it as ADHD.

How to Choose a Specialist for ADHD Diagnosis?

If someone has ADHD, whether it is an adult or a child, they are going to face problematic situations every day and so, getting them the right treatment is very important. There are a lot of specialists that you can go to for getting yourself or your kid diagnosed.

- **Primary Care Doctor** – The first option that is open in front of you is your primary care doctor or general practitioner. They will perform basic diagnosis, and depending upon the situation, they might either refer you to some psychiatrist/psychologist, or they can even prescribe medications.
- **Psychiatrist** – A psychiatrist is a highly trained medical professional in the scope of mental health. They are definitely one of the best people to help you with ADHD diagnosis and prescribe the right meds. They can even

hallmark symptoms of ADHD. But just to give you an idea, some of the factors that the specialist takes note of are as follows –

- **What is the severity of the symptoms?** – If someone has to be diagnosed, then the symptoms that they are having should be severe enough to hamper their life to a great extent. It applies to both children and adults. If you see people who have already been diagnosed with ADHD, you will notice that multiple facets of their life have been gravely affected because of ADHD, and this includes their personal relationships, work, and even financial responsibilities.
- **Do the symptoms show themselves at a particular time?** – If you indeed have ADHD, then the symptoms will pop up in multiple settings and not just in one place. You will face symptoms at the workplace, at home, and even when you are out on a date. It is probably not ADHD if you are facing the symptoms at only one place or one time of the day.
- **When was the first time you noticed the symptoms?** – This is another very important thing to take note of in the diagnosis of ADHD. In the case of ADHD, the symptoms generally start appearing the childhood years. In some cases, people get diagnosed later on when they reach adulthood. Also, if you are an adult, then the therapist might help you trace your current

52

concentration that not only happen in ADHD but in a whole lot of other problems as well. This is why ADHD can be confused with a lot of other medical problems leading to a wrong diagnosis. It is also confused with certain emotional problems and learning disabilities just because there is an overlap in the symptoms. The problem with the wrong diagnosis is that the affected person will then not receive the treatment they deserve or require to cure their actual problem. So, keep in mind that just because your symptoms match with that of ADHD, it doesn't mean that it is ADHD. A thorough diagnosis aided with a properly researched assessment by a specialist is necessary to conclude it as ADHD.

Factors That Are Looked Into

Like I told you earlier, the specialist might you a set of questions that will help him/her to make a proper diagnosis. Every person displays different symptoms when it comes to ADHD. So, in order to make a proper diagnosis, there are different things that have to be considered by the professional and set the criteria accordingly. You should also promise yourself that you are going to be as honest as you can while answering the questions of the specialist; otherwise, the diagnosis will not be accurate.

In short, if someone has to be diagnosed with ADHD, they will have to show strong symptoms. These symptoms are a combination of inattention, impulsivity, and hyperactivity. They are known as the

Chapter 4: Diagnosis of ADHD

Have you not been able to finish any work this week?
Do you keep losing your house keys all the time? Are
you feeling terribly disorganized in your life? As you
know, from Chapter 2, all of these symptoms
definitely point to ADHD. But you also have to keep in
mind that ADHD is much more than these symptoms
alone. So, never jump to any conclusions before you
visit a specialist. If you think about the different
symptoms of ADHD singularly, you will realize that
they are not really that abnormal. Feeling restless or
forgetting things is very common. Even if your
distractibility has reached chronic levels, it doesn't
mean that you have ADHD.

The problematic part is that ADHD cannot be
diagnosed through any physical or medical test. If you
want to know whether you or your child is suffering
from ADHD, you have to visit a specialist or a health
professional who performs such a diagnosis. They
implement a lot of different psychological tools to
predict whether you have ADHD or not. They might
ask you about your past problems or even the present
ones, and you have to answer them honestly; they
might even make a checklist of symptoms for you or
prescribe some medical examinations that will help in
ruling out certain other causes that might be behind
those symptoms.

A proper diagnosis is very important because there
are several symptoms like hyperactivity and loss of

where they declared that only five percent of ADHD kids were benefitted from eliminating sugar from the diet, and most of these kids either had food allergies or were quite young.

- In 2005, an article by Dr. Ruff was published in Clinical Pediatrics, where the term 'epidemic of modernity' was given to ADHD (Ruff, 2005). The article mainly focused on how the development of the brain in kids is affected by the type of life we lead today and the TV shows and video games that kids are exposed to. It was also mentioned that when kids are so into a fast-paced life on the outside, classroom teaching appears to be quite slow to them, and so, they start to treat their academic life with the same urgency that they display in the outside world.

researchers had also concluded that ADHD could not be caused by lead exposure alone, and that lead is only one of the harmful chemicals to cause the symptoms of ADHD in humans. We can also say that a diagnosis of ADHD is not certain by increased lead exposure, but it can definitely be of some help in finding out the actual reason behind the symptoms.

Other Factors That Might Lead to ADHD

In this section, we are going to discuss various factors that might cause ADHD other than the ones already mentioned above.

- A study was conducted to find out whether ADHD can be caused by utero exposure to alcohol and smoking, and the research found that these are indeed risk factors of ADHD (Rosalind J. Neuman, 2007).
- Another study pointed out that preterm birth or babies who are born prior to their delivery date are also at risk of developing ADHD when they grow up (K. Lindstrom, 2011).
- There was a point of time when it was believed that symptoms of ADHD could be reduced if children were made to stop consuming food additives and refined sugar. And so, any food that contained preservatives, sugars, colorings, or artificial flavorings were not given to children. But NIH or National Institue of Research did a conference in the year 1982

- Lastly, BPA or Bisphenol A is another chemical that you should be aware of. It is present in several containers and even food cans, and it is mainly an epoxy resin. Those plastic containers you use at home often contain BPA, and they are even found in certain products made from paper. However, these days you will get several alternative options that are BPA-free.

The participants in the initiative made by LDDI were tested for these toxins. There were a total of 89 chemicals that were studied. Every participant in that listed tested positive for at least twenty-six of those harmful chemicals. Scary, isn't it?

A study was performed by the University of Calgary in 2015 that found that some zebrafish were hyperactive, and this symptom could be traced back to chemicals like BPA and BPS, both of which are present in plastic. But did you know that zebrafish is very important in the studies of embryonic brain development of humans? Yes, and the main reason behind this is that about 4/5th of the genes are common between humans and zebrafish. Moreover, the processes and stages of development are also similar. Since BPS and BPA exposure to these fishes showed negative results in terms of brain developments, the findings of the study proved to be a smoking gun.

Another study that was conducted in the year 2015 showed that ADHD could also be caused by increased exposure to lead (Joel T. Nigg, 2015). But the

chemicals on an everyday basis in the most commonplace areas, and these chemicals have the ability to damage the brain. And here are some of those common chemicals that are harmful –

- Do you know what materials like Scotchgard and Teflon are made of? They contain a particular type of chemical known as PFC or perfluorinated compounds. The main function of these compounds is that they do not allow the food to stick to pans, cooking utensils, carpets, or even curtains.
- Next, we come to another range of harmful chemicals that are easily found in household chemicals, and these are – PBDEs or polybrominated diphenyl ethers. They are found in bedding, furniture, and even clothing items. Their main function is that of a fire retardant.
- The third compound on this list is something that you will get in your personal care products – triclosan. It is found in toothpaste and soaps, and many other items as well. It protects you from harmful bacteria and is itself a harmful chemical.
- The next chemical that I am going to name is already very well-known as being harmful – phthalates. They help to make things pliable and soft, and they are present in a lot of rubber-based and plastic materials like raincoats, bottles, toys, and so on. You will also get them in shampoos and soaps.

why the frontal lobe of the human brain is so extensively researched with respect to ADHD.

Can Pollution and Toxins Cause ADHD?

A scientific research was conducted to find out whether there is a link between disorders like autism and ADHD with that of being exposed to everyday chemicals. The research showed that some kind of link is present and that chemicals in toothpaste or other products related to personal care, cleaning products, flooring, and even foods can contribute to causing ADHD. Moreover, the various systems in our body are still in the stage of development when we are infants, and that is when the human is most vulnerable to these chemicals. The overall physical health of the child and its brain can have a lifelong impact if serious toxins are exposed to important regions of the body when the baby is in a fetal stage. These toxins are known to negatively affect the course of normal brain development in children.

A report was launched by the LDDI or the Learning and Developmental Disabilities Initiative regarding the fact that learning disabilities in humans can occur as a result of certain toxic chemicals. This report was published in the year 2010. In this report, it has been mentioned that people are affected by chemicals even if they are not living somewhere that is right next to a dumping yard or factory. We are exposed to harmful synchronized fashion. But a dopamine deficiency prevents that from happening. So, even if one among these four regions or all four regions has a problem with dopamine, then ADHD might occur. There is, however, no concrete proof regarding which part of the brain is responsible for ADHD symptoms. More clinical trials and experience are required to say anything specifically. The quality of ADHD treatment will improve only when the understanding of these neurochemicals increases.

NAMI or National Institue of Mental Health had published a study in which they were able to pinpoint a particular part of the brain that is affected by ADHD (Philip Shaw, 2007). The part of the brain that is responsible for helping you stay attentive displays thinner tissues in those who have ADHD. But the study also concluded something positive, and that is – when the children grow up, in some of them, the thinner tissues became normal. And consequently, with an increase in the thickness of the tissues, the symptoms of ADHD also began to subside.

Another observation that has been made so far by scientists is that in a small percentage of children, ADHD shows itself after a brain injury. The injury might be a physical one or even an increased exposure to harmful chemicals (you are going to learn more about that in the next section). Experts have noted that people who were not affected by ADHD previously developed the symptoms after encountering head injuries. It is possibly because of damage caused to the frontal lobe. It is also the reason

- **Basal Ganglia** – Next, we come to that region of the brain, which is mainly responsible for maintaining proper communication between different parts. The basal ganglia can be called a neural circuit in simple terms. Whenever a part of the brain has to relay information to another part, it first comes to the basal ganglia. From there, it is then sent to that part of the brain which needs to be communicated. But when the basal ganglia do not have adequate levels of dopamine, it undergoes a phase that is often referred to as the 'short circuit,' and this is what causes impulsiveness and loss of attention.
- **Limbic System** – Contrary to the other parts, the limbic system is situated in the depths of the human brain, and its main function is the manifestation of emotions. When dopamine is deficient in this region, emotions are no longer stable, and the person suffers from restlessness and loss of attention.
- **Reticular Activating System** – There are more than one pathways in your brain, and one of the most critical relay systems is the reticular activating system. And if this system faces any deficiency in the levels of dopamine, then the instant result is hyperactivity, impulsivity, and inattention.

You also have to keep in mind that proper functioning of the brain is only possible when all of these parts of the brain interact with one another to work in a

However, I hope that one day all of these imaging studies and their findings might lead to the discovery of some technique that will help in the diagnosis of ADHD. But if we are talking about today, then this is still a controversial matter.

Apart from this, there are also several chemical changes that are observed in the brain in a patient who is suffering from attention-deficit hyperactivity disorder. As far as the mental health disorders are concerned, you would be surprised to know that ADHD is, in fact, one of the initial disorders that were related to the reduced amounts of dopamine (an important neurotransmitter). ADHD was also one of the first mental health disorders that actually responded positively to the medicines that were used to treat the deficiency of dopamine. When ADHD is diagnosed in adults or even children, it is found that their levels of dopamine are quite low.

The neurotransmitter activity is gravely affected in four core regions of the brain in ADHD patients, and these functional areas are as follows –

- **Frontal Cortex** – Everything staring from executing something to organizing stuff and maintaining concentration is maintained by the frontal cortex region. Inattention is often caused by a reduction in levels of dopamine in this part of the brain. The executive functions are also affected, and so is the ability to organize.

Another study has also proven that genetics does have a serious role to play when it comes to ADHD. In 2010, children with ADHD were examined, and it was found that the brains of these kids either had duplicated pieces of a certain DNA or completely missing DNA (Nigel M. Williams, 2010). The genetic segments that were studied in this experiment are also speculated to be linked with schizophrenia and autism.

How Does ADHD Affect the Brain?

I have already mentioned earlier that ADHD affects the brain, and in this section, we are going to see how. There are several functional and structural differences spotted in the brain of an ADHD patient. When neuro-imaging of an ADHD brain was performed, it showed that the rate of maturation of the brain is much slower. So, kids who do not have ADHD mature faster than those who have ADHD. Apart from this, the areas of the brain that are responsible for playing a part in ADHD symptoms also show some structural differences, and this has been proven by recent research. According to research, a 5% reduction in size is noticed in some regions of the brain of ADHD patients, namely – basal ganglia, striatum, prefrontal cortex, and cerebellum (Ajay Singh, 2015). Now this structural difference that I have mentioned has been found to be consistent in the patients with ADHD, but this is not enough for the proper diagnosis of any random individual.

patients with ADHD, and this is also correlated to the presence of a particular gene. This gene, when investigated, showed that these changes are temporary. When a child approached adolescence and then adulthood, the brain tissues also undergo developmental changes, and thus, several symptoms either manifest themselves differently or subside.

So, it can be said that in some families, ADHD is definitely passed down from parents to children, and this is reinforced by the fact that 1/3rd of those fathers who were diagnosed with ADHD in their childhood years have a child who also has ADHD. Another evidence that suggests the presence of a link between genetics and ADHD is that the disorder is present in most of the identical twins. Also, since ADHD is not a simple disorder and involves a lot of complex aspects, scientists believe that it is not regulated by only one gene but rather two. As far as the genetic field is concerned, there is a lot left to do to find a piece of solid evidence. But if and when this link is found, it would be of immense help to the specialists to diagnose ADHD, and this, in turn, would help the patients to receive the right line of treatment from an early stage. In fact, since the symptoms vary from one person to another, concrete evidence linking a gene can even make the treatment process easier. An Australian study has even shown evidence that when it comes to identical twins, the risk of developing ADHD is even greater as compared to singletons (Megan R. McDougall, 2006).

Well, in several cases, it has been seen that there is strong evidence of genetics playing a role in causing ADHD. If a family member already has ADHD, then a particular person is already prone to developing it as much as four times higher than anyone else. Several genes are now being investigated by scientists all over the world to find a strong and definite connection with ADHD. The genes that are closely related to dopamine are the ones that are most commonly investigated. This is because a common trait is found in people with ADHD – their dopamine levels are way lower than others who don't have ADHD. Here is a quick fact that you should be aware of – dopamine is a chemical in the brain whose main function is to help a person concentrate on something consistently and regularly. But you should be aware of the myths about ADHD since they tend to outnumber the facts and often guide you in the wrong direction.

In short, even though the researchers have not been able to pinpoint any particular cause for ADHD, they definitely have narrowed down to a number of things that are probably behind it, and genetics is one of them. When brain imaging was done of the patients, it revealed that there were significant differences with those who do not have ADHD. Thus, the cause of ADHD is completely biological, and it is not caused by consuming too much sugar or bad parenting or any other hoax that you heard from your neighbor.

In fact, it has also been noticed in studies that the parts of the brain which are responsible for helping you to concentrate often have thinner tissues in even if you have abused your child, you cannot say that your child got ADHD because of it since it does not spread like that. The child or the person who has been suddenly diagnosed with ADHD was definitely predisposed to the disorder. The seriousness of the ADHD symptoms is affected to some extent by the techniques used by parents during their upbringing. But this does not mean that parental approaches somehow cause ADHD. ADHD is solely biological, and the management of the symptoms becomes easier with these psychological approaches.

Before we go into the different causes behind ADHD, I want to make one point clear, and that is – no one is sure as to what is the exact cause behind this disorder. What people have found out until now is that there are multiple possible reasons behind it, and these reasons might not be the same in everyone. For someone, it might be the genes, whereas, for others, it might be something else. Several assessments of behaviors have been done over the years to improve the understanding of this disorder. The heritability factor has received quite an attention after several researchers providing evidence through their assessments. It has been noticed that the genetic contribution is quite popular in those who are being diagnosed with ADHD.

Can Genetics Cause ADHD?

In this section, we are going to approach the issue of whether ADHD is caused by genetic factors or not.

38

Chapter 3: Causes of ADHD

All the scientific research that has been done until now has confirmed that ADHD is a disorder that affects the brain. In this chapter, you will see how at its very core, a problem in brain development that is passed on genetically is the root cause of this disorder. Most of the cases of ADHD that are brought to light have one thing in common – the brain structure is abnormal, and this happens in the unborn child and manifests itself in different ways once the child is born. Some other things that are noticed include an imbalance in the chemical functioning of the brain, and the messages in the brain are not relayed properly. Another thing worth noticing in al of this is that the drugs that are used in the treatment of ADHD are very effective. They can even minimize the effect of the symptoms on the body and corrects many of the imbalances.

The seriousness of the problem can be handled and managed only if the diagnosis of ADHD is made at the right moment, and appropriate measures have been taken. Bad parenting is never the cause of ADHD, and we have clarified this myth before, but what you need to learn is that sometimes, some parents do not bring up their ADHD kids attending to their special needs, and this is what makes situations worse. In the same way, if the parents follow all the strategies for coping up, things will be better for the child when he/she grows up to be an adult. Having said that, I want to say it again that no matter how bad your parenting is,

remember stuff, it makes them anxious. Moreover, those who are facing sleep problems have to go through even worse situations.

All of the symptoms of ADHD in adults mentioned in this chapter give rise to several personal and professional problems. But these difficulties can be overcome, and you will learn to do that in the latter part of this book. If you want to read about why ADHD happens, the next chapter will give you a lot of information on that.

the right path is in order to go from one point to another. They cannot stay fixated to one thing at a time and jump from one task to another. In this way, nothing is ever completed.

Fatigue

People often overlook the fact that one of the most important symptoms of ADHD is fatigue. I know that you might be surprised by this revelation, but this is actually true, and there are multiple reasons behind this. Firstly, those with ADHD are hyperactive most of the time, and this makes them feel tired. They also suffer from inconsistent sleeping patterns. Secondly, in some people, fatigue results from the constant struggle that they have to engage in to focus on their day-to-day tasks. And thirdly, another reason is the medications prescribed for ADHD, which also makes people feel like they are tired all the time. No matter what the cause is, the main point is that fatigue is a very difficult thing to deal with, and it can make life worse.

Anxiety

I have referred to this term quite a lot in this chapter, but you also need to be aware of the fact that anxiety, in fact, is a direct sign of ADHD as well. People feel that they just keep thinking all the time, and there is no moment of peace in their lives. They get frustrated because they have to keep fighting this constant need to keep moving. This is also the reason why people with ADHD are so restless. Another reason why people get so anxious when they have ADHD is that they forget important things. When they cannot esteem suffers. They start criticizing themselves for even the smallest mistakes. They no longer see things positively, and everything is in a negative light. So, everything starting from impulsiveness to difficulty in focusing contributes to the problem of being hypercritical.

Mood Swings

Adults who have ADHD are quite emotionally unstable. All of us experience impatience and anxiety in our lives, which also manifests themselves in the form of anger. But these emotions are magnified to a greater level in those who are suffering from ADHD. These mood swings also affect their jobs and personal lives. Gradually, they feel demoralized, and as if they can do nothing with the situation. Dealing with ADHD symptoms in life is already a difficult task, and there are numerous challenges that crop up along the way, and so, life, in general, becomes chaotic. When these emotional problems are not tended to, they start accumulating until a final outburst and wreaks havoc in life.

Absence of Motivation

Adults with ADHD often don't feel motivated to do things like others. The root of this problem lies in the fact that these people are not able to focus, and thus, they feel unmotivated to complete the task. Moreover, as you already know, the feeling of being overwhelmed is very common in ADHD adults, and this adds to the feeling of being unmotivated. Most people don't even try to accomplish a task and give up way before that. They can't seem to figure out what impulsive or not is to have a close look at their shopping habits. If a person consistently buys things that he/she hardly needs or even cannot afford in normal situations, then they are making impulsive decisions. It is one of the symptoms pointing in the direction of ADHD. It is because of this symptom of impulsivity that adults with ADHD also have temper outbursts from time to time.

Forget Things Easily

People are quite confused about this symptom because all of us tend to forget things from time to time, but does that mean we all have ADHD? No. But on the other hand, those who have ADHD also show symptoms of forgetfulness. They keep searching for common things like keys or glasses because they keep misplacing them. They can even miss their medical appointments or forget to call back people. The bottom line of all this is that whether forgetfulness is due to ADHD or not, it has quite damaging consequences on people's lives and also harms relationships. The forgetfulness in ADHD adults becomes scary when they have important responsibilities like looking after a child. There have been cases where the parent forgot to pick the child up from school or dance lessons.

Hypercritical

The sense of self-image in adults with ADHD is very bad, and they are very much hypercritical. The main reason behind this is that they are so burdened by the disappointments of not completing work on time or meeting several other personal failures that their self-

Disorganization

People will ADHD feel that their life is chaotic, and even when they have a routine in place, things are not quite organized. They might constantly be searching for that one pair of socks that seem to get lost every other day. They fall behind on their monthly bills. Or, their work desk is always full of clutter. In extreme cases, people also lose their jobs, or their careers suffer just because of their disorganized behavior. They constantly feel exhaustion and are overwhelmed with the growing burden of work that is left unfinished. However, if proper strategies are undertaken, these symptoms can be managed. Every person's needs in the case of ADHD are different, and so careful assessment has to be done regarding which strategies you should use.

Impulsiveness

Now we come to the symptom of impulsivity, which means that adults who are suffering from ADHD take actions before thinking them through. There are multiple ways in which this particular symptom can manifest itself in a person. Also, it is not the same in everyone. Something may be true for you, but it might not be the same for someone else. Some common ways in which this symptom shows itself are – finishing tasks in a rush, doing things or saying stuff that is considered to be inappropriate in social settings, interrupting an important conversation suddenly, and doing things without giving a thought to the gravity of the consequences that are to follow. One of the best ways to identify whether a person is

Hyperfocus

In the previous section, we talked about the difficulties faced by people when it comes to focusing, but the flip side to that is also common in adult ADHD, and that is known as hyperfocus. As you might have guessed from the term, hyper-focusing is a state when the person is so engrossed in the task they are doing that they are simply not willing to look in any other direction. They zero in on that single task with a lot of intensity, and you can also say that it is completely opposite to that of distractibility. People don't even realize how hours have passed by, and they were fixated on that one single task.

Problems with Managing Time

This is another trait of adults suffering from ADHD. They cannot figure out how they can effectively spend their time and complete all the tasks on their to-do list. You will often find people with ADHD procrastinating or consistently missing out on appointments. Some people even forget invitations to parties and weddings. The reaction to time and the perception of time in people with ADHD is quite different from those of others. In simpler words, their thought on the time needed to do a particular task might not be the same as someone else's. Some of the researchers and experts have come up with a special term 'time blindness,' which points to this problem of managing time. And the fact that ADHD makes them easy prey to distraction makes matters worse when it comes to managing time.

driving, managing time, compromise, understanding social cues, and so on.

Symptoms in Adults

When ADHD is diagnosed and treated since childhood years, it becomes easier to manage when they grow up. But at other times, the symptoms go unnoticed, and ADHD is left undiagnosed. It doesn't receive appropriate treatment at the right time, and thus, symptoms put a strain on the everyday aspects of life. In order to ensure proper management of the problem, identifying the symptoms and seeking help from a doctor is mandatory. In this section, I am going to introduce you to some of the common symptoms of ADHD, as seen in adults.

Difficulty in Focusing

One of the most prominent signs of ADHD in adults is the inability to focus. Adults with ADHD cannot seem to concentrate on anything for too long. They are distracted very easily, and even when they are in the middle of a conversation, they find it really hard to keep listening to someone over an extended period of time or make an effort to carry on the conversation. Another sign of difficulty in focusing is when a person misses out important details from a conversation and is not able to keep up with their deadlines. In this book, you will learn about several strategies that you can use to increase your focusing power.

world. They are not even much involved in playing with other kids.

Make Careless Mistakes

Children with ADHD need to be constantly reminded and guided to help them complete their tasks, and even after all of that, they make mistakes that are rather careless. Even if you make a set of instructions for the kid, you will notice that the child is facing problems following those instructions. But just because they are making mistakes doesn't mean they are lazy or do not have the willingness to fulfill their dreams. Kids with ADHD have a tendency to make silly mistakes in subjects like Maths, which might seem rather easy to others.

Not Organized

Being organized is a skill that is required at every age, but with ADHD, staying organized is probably the biggest struggle. This can be noticed even at a young age. Kids often fail to keep track of their activities and tasks. The assignments and projects keep piling up, and prioritizing is something that ADHD kids have trouble with. They have to be constantly kept on a routine by their parents, and by following different strategies since childhood, ADHD becomes manageable by the time these kids become adults.

These were some of the common symptoms that are noticed in ADHD kids, but as the children grow up, you will notice that these kids are often seen to be immature when compared to others of their age. They have trouble with so many aspects of daily life like

Avoidance

All the above symptoms that I have mentioned above leads to a type of avoidance in a kid suffering from ADHD. The kids tend to avoid anything that needs them to wait, focus, or give a sustained mental effort. This includes a lot of things and almost all types of schoolwork. For teenagers, this can also mean household chores, which require extensive physical exertion. Anything that requires cognitive effort is totally off the list when it comes to people with ADHD.

Cannot Play Quietly

ADHD children have the habit of talking excessively, and so they are not able to play quietly. This symptom is also a result of the fidgeting problem. ADHD kids are not inclined towards activities and games that require them to stay quiet for a certain period of time. They are always impatient and have this constant need to move around.

Daydreaming

This is another of the very common symptoms of children who have ADHD. You have to keep in mind that daydreaming is just one of the symptoms of ADHD. You cannot diagnose someone with ADHD just because they were daydreaming because lots of kids do. Daydreaming along is never enough to conclude that a child is suffering from ADHD. But those who do have ADHD and daydream are often found staring out in the distance and lost in their own

Tasks Left Unfinished

You will often find that a child who has ADHD is interested in doing a lot of things, but the problem is, they are not too much inclined towards finishing what they started. Let us say your child has a ton of homework to do, and she starts doing it in the evening. But before she can complete it, she hops on to some other task or starts playing. For others, this might seem a problem that is easy to solve and that the child is doing this because they are not trying hard to focus. But that's not the problem here. The child slowly becomes the jack-of-all-trades, and yet they cannot master any. This even applies to leisure activities. If a child with ADHD starts watching a particular cartoon series, then the chances are that they are not going to finish it and would soon start doing something else.

Absence of Focus

Lack of focus is a symptom of ADHD in children, and it affects every aspect of their lives. Even if you are talking to an ADHD child directly, they might not be able to pay you the attention that is required. When you ask them to repeat what you have just said, it is highly likely that they won't be able to do that because they were not focusing on what you were saying. But here you should remind yourself that not every problem that has an attention deficit symptoms is ADHD. But if your child is experiencing troubles in focusing, then the best way to find that out is through the performance of the child in school. Shorter spans of attention are what cause the absence of focus.

Temper Tantrums

A very common symptom of ADHD in kids is their temper flare-ups. In fact, anger and ADHD really go hand-in-hand. The reason behind this is that children who are suffering from ADHD get stressed even in the most commonplace of situations. And so, they are not able to keep a check on their emotions. You will often notice them having an anger outburst in the most inappropriate situation of all. Also, anyone who has ADHD is already very emotionally sensitive. When the kids go to school, they might have some negative experiences as they are not like the other kids. And as parents, you might not always hear about these experiences your kids have at school. When the child comes back home, they have even more tasks to complete apart from the stress that is already on their minds. So, it is quite natural for the kid to show a temper tantrum because he/she is already quite overwhelmed.

Fidgeting

Fidgeting is related to the hyperactivity factor of ADHD. Whenever a child keeps making restless movements, they are said to have bouts of fidgeting, which is a very common symptom indeed. But parents need to understand that the child is not doing this on purpose. The fidgeting is out of their control, and it usually shows that the child is nervous or under stress, or simply bored. You will also notice your child fidgeting when you ask them to sit in one place for too long.

everyone can see it this way. Moreover, the communication skills of ADHD kids are very poor, and this is also the reason why they come off as self-centered.

Trouble Waiting

The next symptom that we are going to discuss is quite a common one – ADHD kids can never hold the patience of waiting for their turn. This applies to any situation where they have to wait in line. Moreover, if they are asked to wait until someone comes back, even then, they cannot sit in one place and will keep fidgeting.

Interrupting

This symptom can be very annoying because ADHD kids do not understand when they shouldn't speak up and when they should. Suppose there is a conversation happening which does not involve them, they might suddenly speak up, interrupting the conversation. Similarly, if other children are playing games that don't involve them, the ADHD kids might go and interrupt their game. But there are several strategies that can help your child practice self-control. The important thing to understand here is that children with ADHD do not mean any harm, and they do not interrupt willingly. Most of the time, they do not even realize that they are interrupting. And this is mainly because the ADHD kids do not understand when someone is angry with them or even frowning.

Chapter 2: What Are the Symptoms of ADHD?

In this chapter, we are going to talk about the symptoms of ADHD and how it looks in both adults and children. Keep in mind that most of the time, the symptoms vary so much from one person to another that it becomes very difficult to identify ADHD. Some people display elaborate symptoms, while others might show only a few symptoms.

Symptoms in Children

In the first section, we will go through the various symptoms as observed in a child.

Self-Centered

The first symptom of ADHD is that the child often does not show any type of empathy towards others and does not try to understand what other people are going through. They cannot understand the needs of others, and thus, they come across as self-centered. This symptom itself leads to other symptoms, mainly trouble to wait and to interrupt often. But are they really self-centered? Maybe not because most of the notion about ADHD kids being self-centered comes from the fact that they are always involved in extreme self-care. They have a routine that they follow rigidly, and this means they do exercise daily, eat at a specific time, and go to bed early. But all of these things help them handle the condition in a better way, but not who doesn't concentrate at school and keeps running around the house. But people are oblivious to the fact that adults, too, are affected by ADHD, and it amounts to as much as 4% of Americans. In adults, however, the symptom of hyperactivity is not so much prevalent or common as in kids. But even then, adults face a lot of problems in their personal and professional lives because of ADHD. It also severely affects their social interactions.

We will discuss the symptoms in detail in the next chapter, but something that you have to understand is that ADHD does not show itself in the same in adults as in children. That is why so many adults either go undiagnosed or are misdiagnosed. In the case of adult ADHD, all the complex tasks of day-to-day life are hampered, and this includes decision-making, judgments, memory, and initiative. Two of the problems that are often confused with ADHD are depression and anxiety attacks. The reason behind this is the similarity in symptoms.

Whenever an adult is diagnosed with ADHD, you have to understand that the person had ADHD even when they were children. It was either not diagnosed at all due to a lack of proper resources, or it was misdiagnosed as a learning disability. In some cases, these people did not have serious symptoms in their childhood, and that is why they were not diagnosed. Whatever the reason may be, since the problem was not diagnosed as ADHD, it did not receive the treatment it should have.

- ***ADHD is a type of learning disability*** –
  This myth itself is the reason why so many
  people are misdiagnosed. Learning disabilities
  are completely different, and ADHD is not one
  of those. It is true that the symptoms of ADHD
  can hamper learning by lowering the capability
  to focus. Moreover, in some people, ADHD and
  learning disabilities co-exist, which makes
  diagnosis all the more confusing and also leads
  to this myth being so popular.
- ***Kids will outgrow ADHD*** – You cannot
  outgrow ADHD. It doesn't happen like that.
  The development changes in the body of a
  person and changes in brain composition can
  alter the symptoms a bit, but ADHD, at the end
  of the day, is a lifelong condition.

These myths need to be dispelled because it is because
of these misconceptions that there is a delay in proper
diagnosis, and society doesn't take appropriate
measures to accommodate people with ADHD. Since
there are no visible symptoms of this disorder, people
often misjudge it or misdiagnose it. This is because
people do not have any idea as to what they are
talking about. And on top of everything, the
misconceptions only add to the shame and guilt of the
patients. So, accurate diagnosis is very important.

Adult ADHD

Whenever we talk about ADHD, the first image that
pops up in our minds is that of a seven-year-old kid

dopamine, and glutamate change their functioning in people with ADHD, and that is why medication is necessary.

- **_ADHD happens only in children_** – It is true that ADHD is common in children, but when a child is not diagnosed properly, then ADHD is carried onto adulthood. If they are diagnosed with ADHD for the first time when they are adults, it means that they were not diagnosed before. And once they are diagnosed, they will be able to realize that they did have the symptoms in their childhood years, but no one paid heed to them. Moreover, some people may be diagnosed in their childhood, but as they grow up, the symptoms of ADHD might not remain the same and evolve into something different.

- **_ADHD can be cured with the help of medication_** – People often have this misconception that just because they are taking meds for ADHD, it is going to cure them. But that's not how it works. Medication for ADHD does not cure the problem. Instead, it simply helps the person to cope with the symptoms. I hate to break it down to you, but ADHD is a lifelong condition and a chronic one at that. The only thing that makes life easier is by learning different skills and coping strategies. Throughout their lives, they will keep on building several such new skills and keep taking medication to aid the process.

worse. ADHD needs to be treated just like any other health problem. It needs medication and psychotherapy.

- ***ADHD is not a serious problem*** – Many people think that ADHD is not a serious problem and so they don't take the appropriate measures. I will agree with the fact that this mental health problem is not life-threatening, but that doesn't mean you will not get bothered by it. The quality of life of a person is severely impacted when they are diagnosed with ADHD. Substance use disorders and anxiety are two things that come hand-in-hand with the problem. Moreover, even adults need to be constantly reminded of their responsibilities so that they can keep up with their lives. These people have to put in a lot of effort to stay financially stable, and they are almost paranoid at all times because their inattentiveness might cost them their jobs. Even though some measures are taken in educational institutions to accommodate people with ADHD, but when it comes to a work setting, employers are not really willing to cooperate with any delay.
- ***ADHD is not a real health issue*** – This point is also similar to the one we just discussed where ADHD is not taken seriously but here, we take things a step further and deal with the myth where people think that there are no chemical imbalanced in the body due to ADHD. But this is not true because all the important brain chemicals like norepinephrine,

themselves. They constantly keep comparing themselves to others because they do not feel productive enough. They see others and want to feel motivated just like everyone else, but they can't. A sustained mental effort is very important in people with ADHD to help them get the day-to-day things done. They have to be reminded constantly because disorganization in life is a very common symptom of ADHD, and we are going to address this issue in this book. But this doesn't mean that they are lazy. They also want to achieve great things in life, but the effort required by an ADHD person to complete a simple task is way more than anyone else. In fact, answering an email might seem too difficult because they have to focus on it for a certain period of time to compose a reply. But do you know why this myth is so harmful? This myth creates a sense of failure and disappointment in those who are suffering from ADHD. They lose their confidence, and their self-esteem takes a direct hit.

- ***ADHD is the result of bad parenting*** – You will often see the parents of ADHD kids and adults blaming themselves because they think it is their bad parenting that resulted in the problem. But it is not. It is true that when someone is diagnosed with ADHD, a certain structure is necessary for their lives, but if the parents think that scolding their child or blurting out harsh words would solve the problem, it won't. In fact, it can make things misconceptions need to be cleared; otherwise, those who are present in the community will be the ones affected the most. Moreover, these myths are why people cannot access proper treatment or diagnosis on time or worse – they are often misunderstood. So, I really hope this section is going to be helpful to all of you.

- ***Girls cannot get ADHD*** – This is absolutely a myth because girls do get ADHD. But the origin of this myth lies in the fact that signs of hyperactivity in young girls are not often seen compared to boys in whom these signs are so prevalent. So, due to the lack of prominent behavioral issues in young girls, people often think that girls cannot get ADHD and so they are also not evaluated as much as boys. Also, the major consequence of this myth is that the condition of ADHD in girls keeps progressing because most of them are left untreated, and so as they grow up, they face issues like anxiety, mood swings, an antisocial personality, and when they approach adulthood, they face other comorbid disorders as well. So, boys and girls should be treated in the same way when it comes to ADHD; otherwise, we won't be able to provide them with the care and support they deserve and need.
- ***Laziness is a sign of ADHD*** – When people are diagnosed with ADHD, several of them are scolded or taunted for being lazy and this, in turn, leads them to feel bad or guilty about

ADHD section in this chapter, then you will know that ADD is basically an older term. In fact, previously, people did not recognize ADHD as a separate entity, and ADD was used to refer to everything. For decades, no proper diagnosis was made.

The main difference between these two terms lies in the symptoms. The three major symptoms of ADHD are as follows –

- Hyperactivity
- Inattentiveness
- Impulsivity

People who are suffering from ADHD struggle with all the three symptoms, but in some people, trouble focusing is the major problem. These people would have been put in the category of ADD if it was before the year 1994, but today, the diagnosis would be made as ADHD. This type of ADHD is described or referred to by several other terms as well, some of which are inattentive ADHD, ADHD inattentive type, or ADHD without hyperactivity. But the common factor in all of these terms is inattention being the main symptom. You will learn more about the various symptoms of ADHD in Chapter 2.

Debunking Common ADHD Myths

Just like everything else, there are some common myths about ADHD in everyone's minds, and I am going to clear the air in this section. These

- At an average, people are diagnosed with ADHD at the age of 7.
- It is between the ages of three and six that the symptoms of ADHD first start to appear.

Now, here are some other important facts that you should know about –

- All the races are affected by ADHD. However, in the span of 2001-2010, a sudden surge of ADHD was noticed in black girls of non-Hispanic origin, and there was as much as over 90% increase.
- 5.5% of Latino children are affected with ADHD, 9.5% of Black children are affected, and 9.8% of White children are affected.
- About 6.4 million children in America have been diagnosed with this disorder. They are all between the ages of 4 and 17.
- Even though the numbers differ from state to state – about 6.1 % of children in America are under ADHD medication and receiving treatment. But 23% of children in American are not receiving any kind of counseling or medication for ADHD.

ADHD Vs. ADD

You will often see these two terms being used on the internet, but here is something that most people miss – ADHD and ADD are not the same things. They are two different problems. If you read the History of subtypes of ADD were formed because of this list, and they were – ADD without hyperactivity and ADD with hyperactivity.

- Finally, in the year 1987, a revised version was published, and here the term ADHD was used
- Then, in the year 2000, the DSM was released as a fourth edition which also identified three subtypes of ADHD, namely –

  o Predominantly inattentive type ADHD
  o Combined type ADHD
  o Predominantly hyperactive-impulse type ADHD

Facts and Statistics

Before we move into greater details, here are five quick facts about ADHD that everyone should know –

- In a person's lifetime, 4.2% of women are usually diagnosed with ADHD. But the numbers are quite high in men at 13%.
- As compared to women, men are most likely to develop symptoms of ADHD. In fact, there are three times more chances of men developing ADHD than women.
- There is no hard and fast rule that ADHD will happen only in childhood. People in America deal with ADHD even in their adulthood, and statistics show that it is almost 4% of adults who are above the age of 18 that encounter ADHD.

Here is a brief description of the timeline of this disease that will help you understand the history better –

- It was in the year 1902 that ADHD was mentioned for the first time. At that time, it was only defined as a defect in children that affects their moral control and is rather abnormal, and this description was given by Sir George Still, who was a pediatrician.
- Then, it was in 1936 when Benzedrine was approved by the FDA. But immediately in the next year, the medicine was found to display some side effects. When this medicine was given to children, their performance and behavior in school showed considerable improvement. However, these findings were largely ignored at that time.
- In the first edition of the DSM, ADHD was not even recognized in the category of mental disorder. The first edition was published in the year 1952. Then in the year 1968, a second edition was published, and in this one, hyperkinetic impulse disorder was listed.
- By 1955, people started understanding ADHD and its nature, and the drug Ritalin was approved by the FDA. This drug is used even today.
- In 1980 came the third edition of the DSM, and it was here that the term ADD or attention deficit disorder was used for the first time in place of hyperkinetic impulse disorder. Two

14

Chapter 1: What Is ADHD?

This is an introductory chapter that will give you the basic concepts of ADHD that you need to know before proceeding to the later chapters of this book. ADHD is an acronym for Attention Deficit Hyperactivity Disorder. As the term suggests, people who have ADHD show impulsive behaviors and are abnormally hyperactive. It is primarily a mental health disorder, and people who experience this cannot sit in one place for too long and cannot focus on the tasks that they are doing. Awareness about this disorder will help people understand it better and seek the help they need. With proper medication and therapy, ADHD can be managed even though it cannot be cured.

History of ADHD

Children are the ones who are most commonly diagnosed with ADHD. It is also referred to as a neurodevelopmental disorder. The age of 7 is when most children are diagnosed with this problem. Another common feature that has been noticed is that it is the boys who are more commonly seen to have this problem as compared to girls. Symptoms might be noticeable in adults as well. Initially, ADHD was not referred to by this term but by a different term – hyperkinetic impulse disorder. After that, it was classified under the umbrella term of mental disorder by the APA or American Psychiatric Association towards the latter part of the 1960s.

addictive effect on the patients. Apart from medicines, behavioral therapy should also be done. When an ADHD patient moves into adulthood, other therapies like psychoeducational therapy and couple therapy provide effective results.

I am thankful to you for choosing this book out of the several options in the market. I tried my best to make this as informative as possible, and so I sincerely hope that you enjoy it.

- It has been found that ADHD is genetic. Concrete evidence to the causes of ADHD has not been found, and it has not been found out clearly as to how this disorder is passed, but the chemical composition of the brain is altered.
- There are several other disorders that co-exist with ADHD, and this makes the diagnosis of the problem quite confusing. People might have behavioral and learning disorders, along with having ADHD.
- The proper diagnosis of ADHD is important if you want the person to recover and lead a normal life. Diagnosis in the childhood years makes adulthood easier because the child learns the coping strategies in the early years, and by the time they are adults, they become an expert at managing their symptoms. The earlier the treatment is provided to a person, the lesser is the chance of the behavioral problems going out of hand.
- There are no laboratory or psychological examinations that help in finding out whether a child has ADHD or not. The method of diagnosis is solely based on a series of conversations and other achievement and IQ tests.
- Proper medication really proves to be helpful in the case of ADHD because they help in lowering the effect of the symptoms. Another thing to keep in mind is that the medicines that are prescribed in ADHD do not have any

People who suffer from ADHD not only have to deal with several behavioral problems but also learning disabilities. All of these symptoms together make up the problem of ADHD. If someone is facing only learning difficulties, it might not be due to ADHD. Also, you have to keep in mind that both these classes of symptoms have to be dealt with differently because the strategies you need to manage behavioral symptoms is not the same as learning difficulties.

In this book, you will get a summary of all the things that humankind has learned about ADHD so far. Apart from that, you will also get detailed information on various aspects of ADHD, as collected from several medical researches and reports. The symptoms of ADHD, as seen in children, are not the same when these same people move into adulthood. I will discuss the symptoms of both children and adults separately.

Some of the very important points that will be elaborated in this book are as follows –

- In the childhood years, ADHD is a very serious mental health disorder and is often overlooked. According to statistics, the disorder is more commonly seen in boys than that in girls.
- ADHD does not cure by itself when a child moves into adulthood. The symptoms might manifest themselves in a different way, but the disorder itself is carried on. It is a lifelong problem.

numbers in boys as compared to girls. In the beginning, it was believed that as the child grows up, the symptoms of ADHD will go away on their own, but now, researchers and psychiatrists understand the fact that ADHD is not a temporary condition but a lifelong one. The symptoms can definitely be managed, but they still persist in some form or the other in adulthood.

There are several proven strategies and mental tools mentioned in this book that will not only help you navigate your life but also improve your management skills. If you are someone who is dealing with ADHD yourself or if you have a family member who has this problem, then this book will help you in several ways moving forward. Building the life that you always wanted will seem possible now that you have the required skillset.

People are not only beginning to understand this problem better, but there have been several advances in terms of treatment of this disorder. In this book, I aim to give my audience a better understanding of how ADHD affects the life of a person and how these symptoms can be managed with a little bit of effort.

But I want to stress on the fact that you should not consider this book as a substitute for seeking proper treatment. This book is more of an aid to the diagnosis and line of treatment followed by a certified physician. I am sure by the end of this book, I will be able to answer several questions that pop up in people's minds.

Introduction

Congratulations on purchasing *Thriving With ADHD Workbook: Guide to Stop Losing Focus, Impulse Control and Disorganization Through a Mind Process for a New Life,* and thank you for doing so.

The following chapters will discuss every aspect of ADHD and how you can lead a productive life with it. The common symptoms in adults, who are dealing with ADHD, are irritability, chronic lateness, and impulsiveness in decisions. If you have to live with all of that for your entire life, then it can definitely be overwhelming, but in this book, you will learn how you can make it seem less of a burden. You will discover several skills that are required in an ADHD patient so that they can mitigate the symptoms and lead a better life.

Before we move into the chapters, I want to clarify something at the beginning of this book – ADHD is not the same as ADD. In previous years, when much research had not occurred on ADHD, it was known by different names, and ADD is one of them. I have given a detailed comparison between these two in Chapter 1. Even though the occurrence of this disorder was found out quite a while ago, it started occurring in greater frequency only now. The different problems that are seen, along with ADHD, include emotional and behavioral disorders and learning disabilities. They cannot spell properly or read a passage. Another thing that is seen is that ADHD is found in greater

Make Decisions Within a Time Limit	120
Don't Over-Commit	121
Your To-Do Lists Should Not Be Too Long	121
Limit Your Distractions	122

Chapter 10: ADHD Anger Management Tips
124

Know What Makes You Angry	124
Take Care of Yourself	125
Take Breaks	126
Think About the Consequences	127
Always Remain Positive	128
Learn to Express Yourself in Other Ways	129

Conclusion	**131**
References	**135**

CBT 73

Chapter 6: Living With ADHD 75

Binge Eating 75
Anxiety 79
Substance Abuse 82
Sleep Problem 83
Stress 85

Chapter 7: How to Sharpen Your Memory When You Have ADHD? 88

What Is Working Memory? 89
When Do We Use Working Memory? 90
Tips to Boost Working Memory 92
Top Strategies for Improving Overall Memory 97

Chapter 8: What Should You Know About the ADHD Diet? 102

What Is ADHD Diet? 102
Sample Meal Plan 107
Best Foods for the ADHD Diet 108
Protein & Complex Carbs 108
Vitamins & Minerals 110
Omega-3-Fatty Acids 112

Chapter 9: Tips to Make Your Life More Organized 114

Throw Out What You Don't Need 114
Maintain a Planner 116
Organize Your Finances 118
Prioritize Your Happiness and Health 119

Impulsiveness	32
Forget Things Easily	33
Hypercritical	33
Mood Swings	34
Absence of Motivation	34
Fatigue	35
Anxiety	35

Chapter 3: Causes of ADHD — 37

Can Genetics Cause ADHD?	38
How Does ADHD Affect the Brain?	41
Can Pollution and Toxins Cause ADHD?	45
Other Factors That Might Lead to ADHD	48

Chapter 4: Diagnosis of ADHD — 50

Factors That Are Looked Into	51
How to Choose a Specialist for ADHD Diagnosis?	53
Diagnostic Challenges	55
Step-By-Step Guide to Diagnosing ADHD	58
Social, Academic, and Emotional Functioning Assessment	58
Clinical Interviews	61
Medical History and Physical Exam	62

Chapter 5: Treatments for ADHD — 64

What Are the Medications Used in ADHD?	64
Stimulants	65
Non-Stimulants	67
Can Therapy Help?	71
Psychoeducation	72
Behavior Therapy	72

Table of Contents

Introduction	**8**
Chapter 1: What Is ADHD?	**13**

History of ADHD	13
Facts and Statistics	15
ADHD Vs. ADD	16
Debunking Common ADHD Myths	17
Adult ADHD	22

Chapter 2: What Are the Symptoms of ADHD?
24

Symptoms in Children	24
Self-Centered	24
Trouble Waiting	25
Interrupting	25
Temper Tantrums	26
Fidgeting	26
Tasks Left Unfinished	27
Absence of Focus	27
Avoidance	28
Cannot Play Quietly	28
Daydreaming	28
Make Careless Mistakes	29
Not Organized	29

Symptoms in Adults	30
Difficulty in Focusing	30
Hyperfocus	31
Problems with Managing Time	31
Disorganization	32

nature of this work, the Publisher is exempt from any responsibility of actions taken by the reader in conjunction with this work. The Publisher acknowledges that the reader acts of their own accord and releases the author and Publisher of any responsibility for the observance of tips, advice, counsel, strategies, and techniques that may be offered in this volume.

© Copyright 2020 by Gerald Paul Clifford. All right reserved.

The work contained herein has been produced with the intent to provide relevant knowledge and information on the topic on the topic described in the title for entertainment purposes only. While the author has gone to every extent to furnish up to date and true information, no claims can be made as to its accuracy or validity as the author has made no claims to be an expert on this topic. Notwithstanding, the reader is asked to do their own research and consult any subject matter experts they deem necessary to ensure the quality and accuracy of the material presented herein.

This statement is legally binding as deemed by the Committee of Publishers Association. Another body binding it legally is the American Bar Association for the territory of the United States. Other jurisdictions may apply their own legal statutes. Any reproduction, transmission, or copying of this material contained in this work without the express written consent of the copyright holder shall be deemed as a copyright violation as per the current legislation in force on the date of publishing and the subsequent time thereafter. All additional works derived from this material may be claimed by the holder of this copyright.

The data, depictions, events, descriptions, and all other information forthwith are considered to be true, fair, and accurate unless the work is expressly described as a work of fiction. Regardless of the

Thriving ADHD Workbook

Guide to Stop Losing Focus, Impulse Control and Disorganization Through a Mind Process for a New Life

Gerald Paul Clifford